Handbook of

NITROUS OXIDE
AND OXYGEN
SEDATION

Handbook of

NITROUS OXIDE
AND OXYGEN
SEDATION

MORRIS S. CLARK, DDS, FACD

Professor, Oral and Maxillofacial Surgery
Director of Anesthesia
Department of Surgical Dentistry, School of Dental Medicine
Professor of Surgery, School of Medicine
University of Colorado Health Sciences Center
Denver, Colorado

ANN L. BRUNICK, RDH, MS

Chairperson and Professor
Department of Dental Hygiene
University of South Dakota
Vermillion, South Dakota

THIRD EDITION

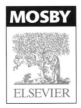

MOSBY

ELSEVIER

11830 Westline Industrial Drive
St. Louis, Missouri 63146

HANDBOOK OF NITROUS OXIDE AND OXYGEN
SEDATION, THIRD EDITION

ISBN: 978-0-323-04827-9

Notice

Knowledge and best practice in this field are constantly changing. As new research and experience broaden our knowledge, changes in practice, treatment and drug therapy may become necessary or appropriate. Readers are advised to check the most current information provided (i) on procedures featured or (ii) by the manufacturer of each product to be administered, to verify the recommended dose or formula, the method and duration of administration, and contraindications. It is the responsibility of the practitioner, relying on their own experience and knowledge of the patient, to make diagnoses, to determine dosages and the best treatment for each individual patient, and to take all appropriate safety precautions. To the fullest extent of the law, neither the Publisher nor the Authors assumes any liability for any injury and/or damage to persons or property arising out of or related to any use of the material contained in this book.

The Publisher

Library of Congress Control Number 2007935286

Vice President and Publisher: Linda L. Duncan
Senior Editor: John Dolan
Managing Editor: Jaime Pendill
Publishing Services Manager: Melissa Lastarria
Senior Project Manager: Joy Moore
Book Designer: Kimberly Denando

Printed in the United States of America

Last digit is the print number: 9 8 7 6 5 4 3 2 1

Working together to grow
libraries in developing countries

www.elsevier.com | www.bookaid.org | www.sabre.org

ELSEVIER   BOOK AID International   Sabre Foundation

FOREWORD

The rapidly advancing medical technology heralds a new era of painless dentistry. Dentists and their patients are no longer satisfied with merely curing the diseases, but they also want a pain-less treatment, a comfortable ride to the land of health. The comfort of patients is not an added bonus; it has become another end that doctors strive to meet today. In the field of anesthesia, this has been rendered possible with the continual development in nitrous oxide and oxygen sedation. The administration of nitrous oxide and oxygen has been widely established in the medical field for over 160 years. It is proven to be a safe and effective approach, easy to grasp and readily accepted, an art that is truly welcomed in today's modern dental practice.

Just as with China's fast economic growth, advancements in the quality and concept of dental care in China have also been progressing to synchronize with the pace of those in developed countries. Development begins with learning from the best. An excellent textbook, a practical handbook, and a clinical guidebook form the foundation for such learning and self-improvement. The *Handbook of Nitrous Oxide and Oxygen Sedation* is all of those. It is concise, elaborate, and accurate. I wholeheartedly recommend it to dentists, dental hygienists, and other medical professionals who would like to master this state-of-the-art technique and who hold an interest in easing the pain and anxiety of their patients.

Dr. Clark and Ms. Brunick are renowned educators. Since 2006, Dr. Clark has visited China several times, to demonstrate the use of sedation in dentistry. While imparting his wisdom, he has also shown us a fervent passion for his profession and a deep desire to further dentistry in China. Indeed, his effort means much to nurturing our next-generation dental anesthetists. His reputation in the specialty of dental anesthesia stretches beyond the limits of the clinical field, as he has devoted himself to the teaching of this art for numerous years.

As the third edition of *Handbook of Nitrous Oxide and Oxygen Sedation* is going into press, I am filled with utmost honor to be given this opportunity to leave a few words of mine in thanking Dr. Clark for the friendship and his contribution to dentistry in China. I believe this new expanded handbook will continue to be a valued reference in dental anesthesia, and it will also testify to the close collaboration between the two countries.

Guang-yan Yu, DDS, PhD
Professor of Oral and Maxillofacial Surgery
Dean, Peking University School of Stomatology
Beijing, China

PREFACE

It is a great pleasure to present the third edition of *Handbook of Nitrous Oxide and Oxygen Sedation*. It seems such a short time ago that the second edition was being completed. In that time interval, much has happened. Importantly, Dr. Horace Wells, the nitrous oxide pioneer and American dentist who was subsequently recognized as the Father of Anesthesia, was honored with a celebration on the 160th anniversary of his death in Hartford, Connecticut. Also notable is the fact that nitrous oxide education for practitioners worldwide has increased dramatically. Globally, China, Turkey, and India have introduced the use of nitrous oxide/oxygen sedation into their inventory of patient management options. The use of nitrous oxide and oxygen sedation has also found more application in varying disciplines and geographic locations.

We have reviewed the worldwide literature over the past 5 years and included applicable, current articles for reference. We have expanded all areas with emphasis on pediatric management. Additionally, photographs and illustrations have been reworked to enhance certain concepts, particularly in the administration technique.

This edition continues to be written in the direct and concise format consistent with the previous editions to facilitate your acquisition of knowledge and quick reference when questions arise. Over the years, we have had the great privilege of interacting with many people about their experiences with nitrous oxide/oxygen sedation. Our heartfelt thanks go to you, our readers. Without your support, this endeavor would not be possible. We appreciate your comments and welcome your feedback and ideas as we continue to use this type of sedation for effective management of our patients' pain and anxiety.

Morris S. Clark, DDS, FACD
Ann L. Brunick, RDH, MS

ACKNOWLEDGMENTS

We appreciate the tremendous support we have received in preparation for this third edition of the *Handbook of Nitrous Oxide and Oxygen Sedation.*

We treasure the relationships we have with the manufacturers of nitrous oxide/oxygen sedation equipment in the United States and sincerely appreciate their dedication to updating and expanding their products. They are, in alphabetical order, Accutron, Inc., Phoenix, AZ; Matrx by Midmark, Versailles, Ohio and Porter Instrument Company, A Division of Parker Hannifen, Hatfield, PA. In particular, we appreciate consultation from Julie Blaisdell, Mike Lynam, and Eric Shirley.

Our international support is made possible by the following individuals: Dr. Jacek Kowalski, Poland; Ms. Zerrin Bakoglu, Turkey; Drs. Guang-yan Yu and Jack Chen, China; Dr. Alberto Aguillar, Mexico; Dr. Yuzuru Kaneko, Japan; Dr. Carlos Plateroti, Argentina; Dr. James Grainger, Austrailia; Dr. Mark Gillman, South Africa; Dr. Eliezer Kaufman, Israel; Dr. Wolfgang Jakobs, Germany; and Dr. Alok and Rupal Patel, India. We thank these people and Dr. Stanley Malamed of the United States for their advice and encouragement.

Several individuals from the University of Colorado Health Sciences Center deserve thanks for their support. They are Dean Denise Kassebaum, Dr. Donald Kleier, Ms. Debbie Malley, Dr. Mike Savage, Dr. Robert Greer, Mr. Nate Turley, and Dr. Avani Khatri. Special acknowledgement is extended to Dr. Danny Abboud for his significant assistance with this text. Others to thank include Dr. Peter Steinhauer, Dr. Elizabeth Barr, Ms. Angela Clark, and Mr. Gregory Clark.

Individuals from the University of South Dakota that deserve thanks are Mr. Glen Malchow, Mr. Eric Dalseide, Ms. Bev Murra, Ms. Beverly Kennedy, Mr. Dan Schulte, Mr. Jose Quiroga, Ms. Ashley Nelson, Ms. Danielle DeYager-Loftus, Ms. Deb Burnight, Ms. Heidi Nickisch-Duggan, Ms. Margaret Morgan, and Mr. Kevin Brady.

Finally, we would like to offer special thanks to John Dolan, Executive Dental Editor at Mosby, Inc. for his assistance and to Ms. Jaime Pendill, Managing Editor. Ms. Pendill has been an invaluable resource for us and we appreciate her support and understanding as we worked toward a quality final product.

CONTENTS

Part I

INTRODUCTION TO NITROUS OXIDE/ OXYGEN SEDATION

Guidelines for Best Practice

INTRODUCTION TO PRACTICE GUIDELINES

Since its discovery more than 160 years ago, nitrous oxide (N_2O) has been used to provide pain and anxiety relief for patients undergoing surgical procedures with a remarkable safety record.[1,2] Clearly, the safety of nitrous oxide use in early days was related more to the inherent safe characteristics of the drug rather than sophisticated insight. Gardner Quincy Colton (1864–1897), an itinerant professor, documented 193,000 cases with no adverse reactions.[3] Ruben,[4] a Danish researcher, cites 3 million cases in which N_2O/O_2 was used in the dental office with no adverse reactions noted. Niels Bjorn Jorgensen[5] attests to 4 million episodes without complications. More than 24 million surgical procedures are performed each year in the United States,[2] and in a large number of them, nitrous oxide/oxygen (N_2O/O_2) in combination with other drugs is used to facilitate general anesthesia. In addition to its use as a general anesthetic adjuvant, myriad health disciplines use N_2O/O_2 sedation alone as an effective means of alleviating patient anxiety and mild discomfort during ambulatory and outpatient procedures. The dental profession has historically used nitrous oxide/oxygen sedation. That experience culminated in the formation of certain criteria for safe administration.[6] In Langa's classic text initially published in 1968, an attempt was made to provide certain guidelines for nitrous oxide/oxygen administration. Today, there is a keen interest in establishing basic guidelines for practitioners who provide all types of sedation, including nitrous oxide and oxygen. In 2002, the American Society of Anesthesiology (ASA) Task Force generated guidelines that should be of absolute importance to all who administer nitrous oxide. These guidelines are promulgated to assist safe and successful administration experiences and maintain to this tremendous historical safety record far into the future.

CURRENT PRACTICE GUIDELINES

The ASA developed guidelines for best practice entitled "Practice Guidelines for Sedation and Analgesia by Non-Anesthesiologists." The document, published in *Anesthesiology*,[7] serves as the overriding policy for defining and directing the trends and practice of N_2O/O_2 administration into the foreseeable future.[7] The guidelines are meant to direct those who are not specialists in anesthesiology, and they are mandatory for nonanesthesiologists practicing in hospitals (e.g., physicians, dentists, podiatrists). They are clearly useful and set the standard of care for future practice. The guidelines will be referred to throughout this text, because they represent an extensive evaluation and a synthesis of expert opinion by numerous academic and clinical anesthesiologists across the United States.

In addition to the ASA guidelines, the American Academy of Pediatrics (AAP) and the American Academy of Pediatric Dentistry (AAPD) have conjointly updated practice guidelines for the sedation of pediatric patients because of its increased use in nontraditional settings.[8] This document, published in *Pediatrics* in December 2006, is titled "Guidelines for Monitoring and Management of Pediatric Patients During and After Sedation for Diagnostic and Therapeutic Procedures: An Update."[8] Similar to the ASA guidelines, this document refers to those practices and procedures that will promote the safe use of sedation for the pediatric patient. This text will also refer to these recent guidelines.

In October 2002, the American Dental Association (ADA) House of Delegates adopted the "Guidelines for the Use of Conscious Sedation, Deep Sedation and General Anesthesia for Dentists."[9] Included in these guidelines for the first time is the term *titration* and its definition. Although the guidelines are not intended for anxiolysis produced by N_2O/O_2 alone, they do refer to the use of N_2O/O_2 in combination with other pharmacologic methods when moderate sedation is intended. An ADA policy statement associated with this topic is currently being proposed for revision and is likely to include additional information about drug pharmacology and understanding the levels of sedation.[10]

This text focuses on the use of N_2O/O_2 in an ambulatory setting. Much of the literature relates to the use of N_2O as an adjunct anesthetic in the operating room for general anesthesia; therefore, reference will be made to articles in the literature in that setting. However, when N_2O/O_2 is used in the ambulatory setting, it is used for minimal periods of time and with lower-percentage concentrations. The ASA Practice Guidelines for Sedation and Analgesia by Non-Anesthesiologists do not address minimal sedation or anxiolysis, which is the administration of N_2O in concentrations less than 50%. The guidelines exclude minimal sedation, because at this level of sedation, the risks are minimal and adverse effects are negligible. Occasionally, the practitioner may apply N_2O in concentrations greater than 50%. For this reason, we will also address the ASA and AAP/AAPD recommendations for moderate sedation, because this is the category in which administration of N_2O in concentrations greater than 50% is placed. The guidelines recommend that the practitioner be responsible for the patient at the intended level of sedation and the next (deeper) level of sedation, because there are specific levels of responsibility for the nonanesthesiologist when a patient is sedated at deeper levels. This concept is clearly based on the practitioner being thoroughly educated and trained, thereby increasing the safety margin for the patient. In this edition of the text, we include recommendations for managing moderate sedation and management of the airway.

VIRTUES OF NITROUS OXIDE

Nitrous oxide is notable because of its impeccable safety record, which has withstood the test of time longer than any other drug. For the patient, N_2O/O_2 provides pain control and anxiety relief that is quickly and easily reversed. It is virtually completely eliminated from the body when its use is discontinued. For the practitioner, the drug is easily titrated to the level required for the procedure while accommodating the patient's physiologic and psychologic needs. When used as a mild analgesic and sedative, N_2O is administered with oxygen from safe, modern equipment that allows no more than 70% N_2O and no less than 30% O_2 to be delivered at any time. The patient is mildly sedated and responds to verbal commands. Protective defenses such as the cough and gag reflexes remain intact; clinical action and elimination are rapid. Recovery is complete within a short time. Few side effects are associated with N_2O, provided the operator uses updated equipment and an appropriate technique. Most often, patients' negative experiences with N_2O have been caused by oversedation by the operator. To that end, this text will emphasize the titration aspect of the administration technique. N_2O/O_2 sedation is still simple and safe to use. N_2O/O_2 sedation may not provide the desired results for all practitioners, nor will it be an option for all patients. However, it continues to maintain its position for effective pain and anxiety management.

REFERENCES

1. Smith WDA: *Under the influence: a history of nitrous oxide and oxygen anesthesia*, Park Ridge, Ill, 1982, Wood Library, Museum of Anesthesiology.
2. Kole T: Assessing the potential for awareness and learning under anesthesia, *J Am Assoc Nurse Anesth* 61:571, 1993.
3. Chancellor JW: Dr. Wells' impact on dentistry and medicine, *J Am Dent Assoc* 125:1585, 1994.
4. Ruben H: Nitrous oxide analgesia in dentistry, *Br Dent J* 132:195, 1972.
5. Jorgensen NB: *Sedation, local and general anesthesia in dentistry*, ed 2, Philadelphia, 1985, Lea & Febiger.
6. Langa H: *Relative analgesia in dental practice: inhalation analgesia and sedation with nitrous oxide*, Philadelphia, 1976, WB Saunders.
7. ASA Task Force.: Practice guidelines for sedation and analgesia by non-anesthesiologists, *Anesthesiology* 96(4):1004, 2002.
8. AAP/AAPD Clinical Report: Guidelines for monitoring and management of pediatric patients during and after sedation for diagnostic and therapeutic procedures: an update, *Pediatrics* 118(6):2587, 2006.
9. American Dental Association: *Guidelines for the use of conscious sedation, deep sedation, and general anesthesia for dentists*, ADA House of Delegates, October 2002, American Dental Association.
10. American Dental Association Policy Statement: *The use of conscious sedation, deep sedation and general anesthesia in dentistry*, October 1999 and currently under revision, 2007.

History and Evolution of N$_2$O/O$_2$ Sedation

*The only thing new under the sun is the history we have not
read...* Anonymous

$\backsim \frown$

In this era of sophisticated medicine and advanced technology, it is easy to forget what early medical scientists went through to advance standard practices such as N$_2$O/O$_2$ sedation. What these scientific pioneers accomplished while experimenting with unknown, potentially dangerous materials and primitive equipment was courageous. They often sacrificed their own health and safety for scientific advancement. It is because of the bravery of these early medical explorers that we can provide safe and effective analgesia and anesthesia today. The history of nitrous oxide, which cannot be completely captured in this chapter, is rich and enjoyable and is highly recommended reading.

I. HISTORICAL PERSPECTIVES

A. Discovery of N$_2$O and O$_2$
1. The discovery of both N$_2$O and O$_2$ is credited to the English gentleman, Sir Joseph Priestley.
2. The actual discovery dates of these gases are somewhat in question because of Priestley's own uncertainty about what he had discovered. The periods cited in the literature vary from 1771 to 1777.[1] During this time, he repeated several experiments that ultimately resulted in the gases we know today as N$_2$O and O$_2$.
3. Priestley experimented with nitrous air—a mixture of iron filings, sulfur, and water. The end product was a residual gas with considerably less volume than the original nitrous air. He called this "dephlogisticated nitrous air," which is now known as nitrous oxide.[1]
4. During his experiments with nitrous air, Priestley became aware of another gas, which he termed "good air." He found this air to be "fit for respiration," and he titled this discovery "dephlogisticated air," which is now known as oxygen.[1]

B. Inhalation of N$_2$O
1. Humphrey Davy, at the age of 21, was interested in the field of medicine. Although N$_2$O gas was allegedly etiologic to many diseases and deadly conditions, Davy ignored the warnings and, in England in 1798, became the first to chronically inhale pure N$_2$O.
2. Instead of incurring some dreadful plight, Davy found the experience very pleasurable; he became euphoric and felt like laughing. He continued his experiments, saying they produced the "most voluptuous sensations." Other descriptions of his experiences with N$_2$O included "ideal existence" and "overwhelming joy."[2] Davy published the results of his experiments in booklet form in 1800.

3. It was when Davy experienced diminished pain from a toothache while using N_2O that he began to believe it could affect pain sensations. This was the first indication of the anesthetic properties of the gas. Davy had no idea of the significance of this experience.

4. For the next four decades, experiments with N_2O continued, but not in the medical field. Nineteen-year-old Samuel Colt (of firearm fame), posing as a physician, began sporting street corner sideshows featuring N_2O. These shows were touted as a way for young people to enjoy evening entertainment during which they could "laugh, sing, speak, or fight."[3] N_2O use became the trendy activity at social events and in university settings (Figures 2-1 and 2-2). It was the featured demonstration at many lectures.

5. The anesthetic value of N_2O first realized by Davy was not pursued.

C. **Medical world ignores N_2O as potential anesthetic**
    1. During the early nineteenth century, although reckless use of N_2O continued, the medical community was hungry for pain relief. Surgical procedures often resulted in death of

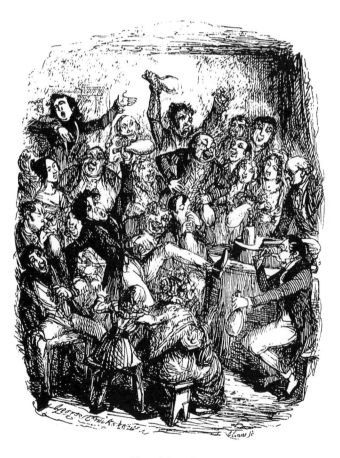

Laughing Gas.

Figure 2-1 "Laughing Gas." *(From Scoffern: Chemistry No Mystery, 1839. Courtesy of the Harvard Medical Library in the F.A. Countway Library of Medicine, Boston, Mass.)*

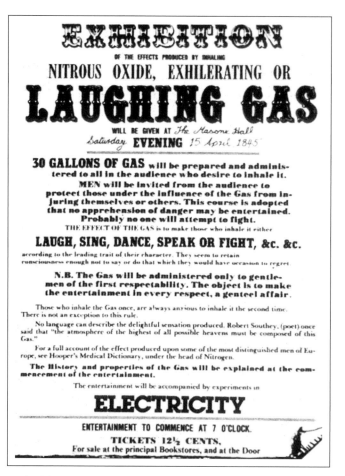

Figure 2-2 Poster advertising a nitrous oxide exhibition. *(From Malamed SF: Sedation, ed 4, St Louis, 2003, Mosby.)*

patients for many reasons. Poor infection control often led to secondary infections, and pain control was desperately needed.

2. The most commonly performed operations were amputations, tooth extractions, and abscess drainings. These surgeries were often completed in less than 90 seconds. During lengthy procedures, patients would succumb to exhaustion and/or shock.

3. The greatest medical advance at that time was the suture. Wounds could be sewn closed rather than cauterized with a hot iron; extremities remaining from amputations did not have to be dipped in a boiling solution to create hemostasis.[3]

4. Rather than face an operation without pain control, patients often committed suicide. Available pain control measures were time-consuming, unpredictable, inconsistent, and at best mildly effective. Several methods were tried:
    a. Brute force to control a patient
    b. Alcohol or opium
    c. Tourniquets or ice

5. Prospective surgical patients were often placed in serious dilemmas—choosing between pure torture and unfathomable pain associated with surgery or living with a disease or condition that would likely result in a slow, agonizing death.

D. The revelation at Dr. Colton's grand exhibition

1. Dr. Gardner Colton, a Columbia University dropout-turned-professor, hosted the Grand Exhibition in Hartford, Connecticut, on December 10, 1844. It was an exhibition to demonstrate the exhilarating effects of inhaling N_2O.[4]

2. Horace Wells, a dentist, was in attendance. As a participant, Wells volunteered to try the gas on stage, believing he would not "make a spectacle of himself." However, that was exactly how Mrs. Wells described his performance.[2]

3. Another participant, a young man named Samuel Cooley, volunteered to inhale the gas in front of the audience. He began to feel the effects of the gas immediately. As he was euphorically jumping around, he struck his leg against a bench, causing a deep, bloody laceration. Cooley was unaware of the extent of the injury and professed that he did not feel any pain.

4. Wells was very intrigued by the apparent nonresponsiveness of Cooley to pain and asked Colton whether a tooth could be removed under the influence of N_2O. Unaware of any analgesic properties, Colton agreed to bring a supply of gas and meet Wells at his office the next day. There Wells breathed the gas himself and had a colleague, Dr. Riggs, extract one of his teeth. Wells exclaimed "the greatest discovery ever made," and "a new era in tooth pulling." Colton taught Wells how to prepare the N_2O and thought of him as a "visionary enthusiast."[4] Figure 2-3 shows a one-of-a-kind portrait of Wells that appears at the Wadsworth Atheneum in Hartford, Connecticut.

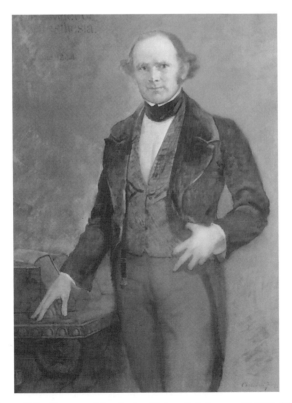

Figure 2-3 Portrait of Dr. Horace Wells, Discoverer of Anesthesia. *(Wadsworth Antheneum, Hartford. Gift of Charles Nöel Flagg. Endowed by C.N. Flagg and Company.)*

E. The Horace Wells experiment

1. Wells used N_2O during extractions on several patients with great success. Anxious to demonstrate this procedure in front of his peers, Wells was allowed to operate in front of several physicians and students in Boston in 1845. As he attempted to remove a tooth, the patient jumped in the chair, leading observers to believe he was in pain. Some time later the patient indicated he did not experience any pain.[4] Unfortunately for Wells, his experiment was deemed unsuccessful, and he was labeled a "charlatan" and a "fake."[5]

2. Wells, in his own writings, indicated that he was obsessed with proving the legitimacy of his techniques. He also alluded to being severely depressed over the debacle in Boston.[5]

3. For the next several years Wells continued to provide anesthesia for surgeons in the area. Dentists began to give attention to the use of N_2O. In fact, advancing dentistry's reputation hinged on the success of extracting teeth with pain relief.[6]

II. EVOLUTION OF ANESTHESIA

A. Ether anesthesia

1. William Morton, a dental student of Wells' and later a physician, was present at the famed event presented by Wells in Boston. Believing that a more potent anesthetic gas was necessary, he began to work with ether.

2. In 1846, Morton performed a surgical demonstration with ether in the Massachusetts General Hospital, later called the "ether dome" (Figure 2-4). Morton's experiment was similar to Wells' in terms of poor success; the patient stated that he felt the procedure as it was performed. However, the demonstration was well received by the audience primarily because of Morton's status as a physician rather than a dentist.[7]

3. Surgical procedures that used ether continued. Other individuals claiming to be the discoverer of anesthesia led Morton to fight for recognition. Morton died tragically in 1848 never having been officially recognized for his accomplishments.

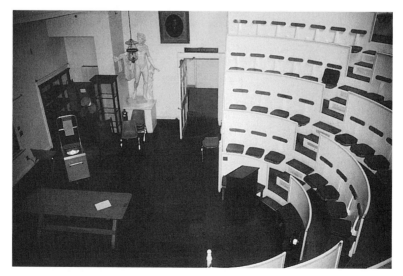

Figure 2-4 The "Ether Dome" present (1997). *(Photo courtesy of Dr. Peter Jacobsohn.)*

B. **Chloroform anesthesia**
   1. In 1847, English obstetrician James Simpson was pleased with the anesthetic properties of ether for his patients. However, he did not like the odor or its potential to induce vomiting. He began to use chloroform as an analgesic for labor pains despite others' claims of significant negative consequences.[6]
   2. Chloroform continued to be a major anesthetic agent into the 1860s and became standard issue to soldiers who, when injured in battle, could self-administer it.[3]

C. **The fight for recognition**
   1. After his failed performance with N_2O as an anesthetic, Wells' whereabouts and mental status were uncertain for a few years. It was very important to him that he prove his credibility and be recognized for his accomplishments. Although the concept of addiction was not recognized at that time, Wells had become a chloroform addict with unpredictable behavior. Inhaling chloroform contributed to his mental decline and, while in a stupor, Wells threw acid on a prostitute in New York City and was imprisoned in 1848. He asked to retrieve some personal items from his home and brought a razor and some chloroform back to his cell. He wrote his last words to his wife and committed suicide by cutting his femoral artery while under the influence of the drug. His suicide on May 30, 1848, ended his life at the age of 33; Wells was unaware of the recognition that would soon be credited to him naming him the "Father of Anesthesia."[5]
   2. The Medical Society of Paris, France, was the first to grant Wells "all the honors of having first discovered and successfully applied the uses of vapors or gases whereby operations could be performed without pain"[4] (Figure 2-5).
   3. In Hartford, Connecticut, every physician had signed a document proclaiming Wells as the primary discoverer of anesthesia.[8]

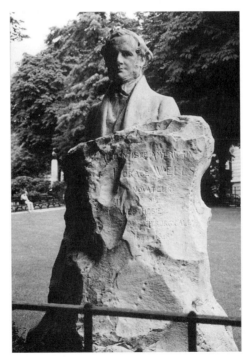

Figure 2-5 Bust of Horace Wells in the Etats Unis Park near the Arc de Triomphe in Paris, France (2002).

4. In 1864, the American Dental Association (ADA) officially recognized him, and in 1870 the American Medical Association (AMA) proclaimed this honor. Reaffirmation was proclaimed by the AMA on the one hundredth anniversary (1944) of the original exhibition, and in the sesquicentennial year (1994), several dental and anesthesiology societies affirmed once again Wells' significant contributions to the health professions.[8] Also in 1994, he was posthumously awarded the Doctor of Dental Surgery degree from the Baltimore College of Dentistry, the first school of dentistry in the United States.

5. In addition, Dr. Leonard F. Menczer led a nationwide petition for a commemorative postage stamp.[9] Unfortunately, despite thousands of signatures, the stamp has yet to be issued.

6. The Horace Wells Club, an organization of dentists and physicians, was formed in 1894 in Hartford, Connecticut, on the fiftieth anniversary of Wells' discovery. They have been meeting annually since its inception to remember this great benefactor and foster the study of anesthesiology. The Horace Wells Club sponsors scholarships for dental students from Connecticut, and they restore and maintain the statue of Horace Wells in Hartford's Bushnell Park (Figure 2-6). They also present an award of merit annually to an individual who has demonstrated leadership and achievement in the field of sedation.[10] Fund-raising efforts sponsored by the Horace Wells Club, the Hartford Medical and Dental Societies, and the Connecticut Dental Association have been held to honor Horace Wells and raise funds to restore Wells' tomb in Cedar Hill Cemetery and support the local suicide prevention organizations (Figure 2-7).

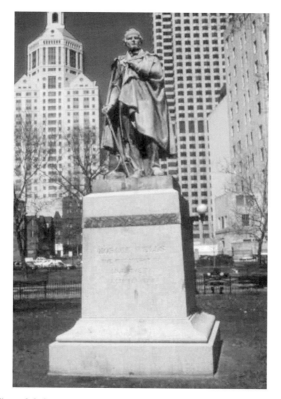

Figure 2-6 Statue of Horace Wells in Bushnell Park, Hartford, Connecticut.

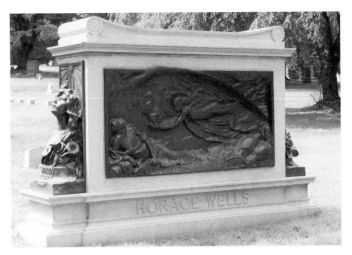

Figure 2-7 Horace Wells' tomb in Cedar Hill Cemetery, Hartford, CT was restored and rededicated in 2004.

D. Resurgence of N_2O

1. The same Dr. Colton who supplied Wells with N_2O in 1844 was responsible for its resurfacing in the early 1860s. Colton insisted that pure N_2O was safe and had an impeccable record of cases to prove it. Between 1864 and 1897, Colton documented 193,000 cases with no fatalities.[6] This began the establishment of its safety record.

2. In 1868, Dr. Edmund Andrews suggested that, when 100% N_2O is used, the blood is not appropriately oxygenated. Andrews added O_2 to the N_2O and claimed one fifth of the volume should be O_2.[2]

3. Also in 1868, Paul Bert developed equipment to deliver both O_2 and N_2O to a patient.[11] He recommended greater atmospheric pressure when N_2O/O_2 was used for human surgeries. However, although his idea was ingenious, it was impractical because of the size and relative immobility of the associated equipment.

E. Twentieth century

1. Dentistry continued to be the primary health discipline to use N_2O. However, except for episodic periods between 1913 and 1938, N_2O use was almost nonexistent. Reasons for this inactivity were unreliable equipment, failure to produce satisfactory results, and lack of knowledge of technique.

2. Cyclopropane was discovered in 1929 and was subsequently used in the clinical setting as a general anesthetic. An excellent anesthetic, it remained the most popular agent for general anesthesia for the next 30 years; its use declined because of flammability issues.[7]

3. Medical residencies in the 1930s included N_2O information in their curricula. Anesthesia became a specialty in 1941.[6] Dr. Harry Langa, an early proponent of N_2O/O_2, began postgraduate dental education in 1949 and trained more than 6000 dentists in N_2O/O_2 sedation. Dr. Langa also published a classic textbook on N_2O inhalation analgesia.[2]

4. Physicians were not satisfied with the availability and effectiveness of intravenous (IV) agents until sodium thiopental (barbiturate) was deemed acceptable in 1935.[7]

5. Anesthesiologists used curare in the 1940s to provide muscle relaxation with light levels of sedation during surgery. When curare was used with N_2O, the incidences of mortality and morbidity were decreased. This combination became the anesthetic of choice for high-risk patients, because it did not threaten the cardiovascular system.[7]

6. The 1940s brought the discovery of lidocaine, a local anesthetic not associated with allergies and other potential medical problems of its predecessor procaine, to dentistry.[12] The popularity and acceptance of local anesthesia temporarily diminished the use of N_2O. When the role of N_2O was revised to assist with the management of anxiety, its popularity began to rise again.

7. The nonflammable anesthetic agent halothane was introduced in 1956,[7] which introduced an entire new era of anesthetic techniques. Halothane was highly regarded in the medical community because of the minimal side effects associated with its use. This offered a great improvement over other general anesthetics at the time. N_2O was used as an adjuvant drug to induce the effects of halothane.

8. N_2O remained functional and was commonly used for general anesthesia as a way to provide rapid induction of other, more potent agents.

9. Dental schools began teaching the concepts of inhalation sedation in the late 1950s and early 1960s. In 1962, the American Dental Society of Anesthesiology established guidelines for teaching pain and anxiety control in dentistry. Today this organization remains at the cutting edge, helping to develop new drugs, techniques, and training for dentists in the area of anesthesia. Also, the International Federation of Dental Anesthesia Societies (IFDAS) is an organization composed of component societies from around the globe. They convene every 3 years to present the latest in scientific data and exchange research findings for the promotion of pain and anxiety control. N_2O continues to be popular in the field of dentistry; approximately 56% of general dentists, 85% of oral and maxillofacial surgeons, and 88% of pediatric dentists use it in their clinical practices.[13,14]

10. Trends followed in other disciplines. Great Britain began the use of N_2O in emergency medicine and for labor and delivery.[15] Podiatry first cited its use in the literature in 1966.[16] Many other health disciplines have begun the use of N_2O/O_2 sedation as a treatment modality for procedures not requiring general anesthesia. See Chapter 15 for more information on the use of nitrous oxide/oxygen sedation in various disciplines.

11. Market predictions showed an increase in the consumption of N_2O through the year 2000 and its use continues to be strong.[17] The popularity of N_2O has waxed and waned over the years; however, it has remained in continuous use longer than any other drug. Despite the advent of other attractive agents, N_2O has never been replaced and has withstood the test of time.

REFERENCES

1. Smith WDA: *Under the influence: a history of nitrous oxide and oxygen anaesthesia*, London, 1982, Macmillan.
2. Langa H: *Relative analgesia in dental practice: inhalation analgesia with nitrous oxide*, Philadelphia, 1968, WB Saunders.
3. Fenster JM: How nobody invented anesthesia, *Am Herit Invent Technol* 12(1):24, 1996.
4. Jacobsohn PH: Dentistry's answer to "the humiliating spectacle": Dr. Wells and his discovery, *J Am Dent Assoc* 125:1576, 1994.
5. Menczer LF, Mittleman M, Wildsmith JA: Horace Wells, *J Am Dent Assoc* 110:773, 1985.
6. Chancellor JW: Dr. Wells' impact on dentistry and medicine, *J Am Dent Assoc* 125:1585, 1994.
7. Kennedy SK, Longnecker DE: History and principles of anesthesiology. In Hardman JG, Limbird LE, editors: *Goodman and Gillman's: the pharmacologic basis for therapeutics*, New York, 1996, McGraw-Hill.
8. Jacobsohn PH: What others said about Wells, *J Am Dent Assoc* 125:1583, 1994.
9. Jacobsohn PH: Remembering Dr. Menszer, *J Am Dent Assoc* 125:1582, 1994.
10. Rosenberg M: Personal communication with 2001 Horace Wells Club Award of Merit winner, October 2002.
11. MacAfee KA: Nitrous oxide. I. Historical perspective and patient selection, *Compend Contin Educ Dent* 10:352, 1989.

12. Malamed SF: Local anesthetics: dentistry's most important drugs, *J Am Dent Assoc* 125:1571, 1994.
13. ADA Survey Center: *1994 quarterly survey of dental practice*, 3rd quarter, ADA News, 1994.
14. Davis MJ: Conscious sedation practices in pediatric dentistry: a survey of members of the American Board of Pediatric Dentistry College of Diplomates, *Pediatr Dent* 10:328, 1988.
15. Baskett PJF, Bennett JA: Pain relief in hospital: the more widespread use of nitrous oxide, *BMJ* 2:509, 1971.
16. Arancia L: Nitrous oxide inhalation analgesia in ambulatory foot surgery, *J Am Coll Foot Surg* 5:111, 1966.
17. Frost & Sullivan, Inc: Anesthesia, gas monitoring markets to grow slightly, top $600 million by 2000, *Anesth Prog* 41:64, 1994.

Chapter 3

Pain and Anxiety Management

A ccording to the American Pain Society (APS), pain is the leading public health problem in the United States and is the most common complaint by people seeking medical care.[1] This organization also cites that pain is the reason why more than 50 million days of work are lost each year.[1] It is estimated that $100 billion are spent in the United States annually for pain-related costs.[1] This economic impact on the nation's population affects all of our citizens directly or indirectly. Statistics also show that as many as 35 million people in the United States avoid the dental office because of their fear,[2] and dental phobia affects 10–12 million people.[3] Fear and pain are interrelated. People will endure severe pain before seeking professional care often because of the fear that is associated with pain.[4] Individuals may find themselves in an emergency situation facing significant problems as a result of not having sought treatment at an earlier time when treatment could have increased the possibility of a favorable outcome.

Managing a patient's pain and anxiety before performing a medical procedure provides an environment that benefits both patient and clinician. Obviously, if you, the clinician, know that your patient is relaxed and comfortable, you can provide better service with less stress (Figure 3-1). Many options are currently available for pain and anxiety relief. Some options in certain situations will prove more advantageous than others. But for many procedures, several methods could be used. In those cases in which assistance in analgesia and anxiolysis would be beneficial, inhalation sedation with N_2O/O_2 should be a primary consideration.

I. MECHANISM OF PAIN

A. Definition

As defined by the International Association for the Study of Pain, "pain is an unpleasant sensory and emotional experience arising from actual or potential tissue damage.[1] The experience includes the perception of an uncomfortable stimulus and the response to that perception."[5]

B. Principles of action

1. The objective of pain is to provide damage protection to tissue by alerting the central nervous system (CNS) before or during a potentially damaging occurrence.
    a. Pain receptors (nociceptors) are the first to receive a stimulus. These receptors are nonspecialized, bare nerve endings that record the occurrence, intensity, duration, and location of the sensation.[6]
2. The theory of pain modulation suggests that impulses are altered along the way by an endogenous opioid system[7] (Figure 3-2).
3. Exogenous morphine binds to an opiate receptor, which accounts for its analgesic properties. Morphine is the drug to which endogenous opiates and other opioid drugs are compared.[7]

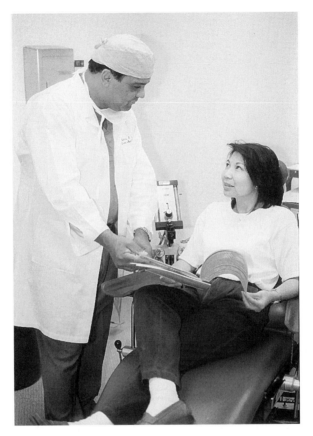

Figure 3-1 Reassuring an anxious patient.

4. Research has attempted to determine the effect of N_2O on the endogenous opioid system. Gillman[8] proposes that analgesic concentrations of N_2O may act directly on the opioid receptor and/or activate the release of endogenous opiates.

5. There is a physiobiochemical relationship between N_2O and opioids. Naloxone hydrochloride (Narcan) can produce reversal effects of opioid drugs. This drug is most commonly used in opioid overdose situations.[9] Oxygen alone will replace N_2O and thereby recover its effects.

6. Endogenous endorphins, enkephalins, and dynorphins have been discovered as substances that bind to the opiate receptors, resulting in pain modulation.[6,7] Activation of the endogenous opioid system can be accomplished by pain and/or stress.[10] Research of the endogenous opioid system continues.

7. Reactions to pain vary from individual to individual and can vary in the same individual from day to day. Many factors can influence pain reactions. Examples of these factors may be categorized as physical, mental, biochemical, psychogenic, social, physiologic, cultural, and emotional.[5] The American Pain Society Task Force on Pain in Infants, Children, and Adolescents suggests that pain is subjective and multifactorial. They suggest that behavioral components are mixed with other factors, including environmental, developmental, and sociocultural factors.[11] In a statement about the assessment and management of acute pain in young people, the AAP and APS state that suffering occurs when pain is overwhelming or chronic.[11]

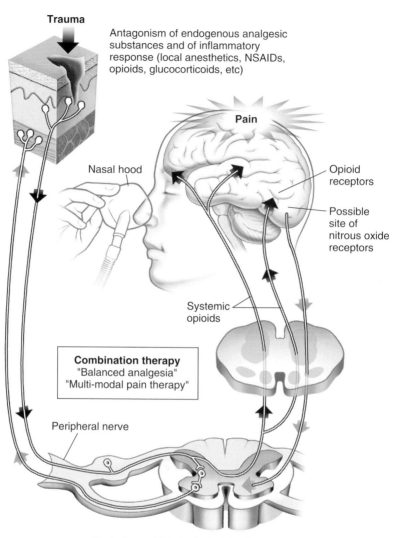

Trauma

Antagonism of endogenous analgesic substances and of inflammatory response (local anesthetics, NSAIDs, opioids, glucocorticoids, etc)

Pain

Nasal hood

Opioid receptors

Possible site of nitrous oxide receptors

Systemic opioids

Combination therapy
"Balanced analgesia"
"Multi-modal pain therapy"

Peripheral nerve

Central neural blockade (epidural/intrathecal local anesthetics, opioids, α_2-agonists)

Figure 3-2 Site of action of various analgesics.

C. **Assessing and measuring pain**
   1. A variety of scales are intended to objectify the levels of pain to allow clinicians to act appropriately and alleviate discomfort. In many cases the scales have been helpful to facilitate self-reporting; however, some have not been useful.[12–15]
   2. A common scale (represented as either vertical or horizontal) depicts pain in equal segments across the continuum from 0 (no pain) to 10 (unbearable). This Visual Analog Scale can be used generally with any age group[15,16] (Figure 3-3). Several other measures have been used; versions of various scales depict a range of facial images from comfortable to painful (Figure 3-4) for visually oriented populations such as children. Numeric scales prove useful when treating chronic pain, because they can

PAIN ASSESSMENT
Pain Rating Scales

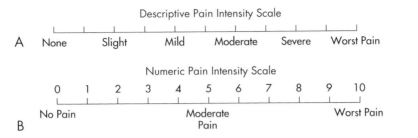

Figure 3-3 Visual analog scales. **A,** Descriptive pain intensity scale. **B,** Numeric pain intensity scale. *(From Mosby's Nursing PDQ, St. Louis, 2004, Mosby)*

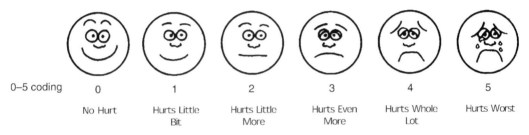

Figure 3-4 Wong-Baker FACES Pain Rating Scale. *(From Hockenberry MJ, Wilson D: Wong's Nursing Care of Infants and Children, ed 8, St. Louis, 2007, Mosby.)*

serve as baseline references over time. Pain scales are deliberately simple to allow people to express themselves when their attention span is decreased and cognitive skills are impacted.

3. Even the simplest attempt to convey understanding of a patient's pain is appreciated. For example, try to use a word for pain from the patient's native language. Some examples are listed in Box 3-1.

4. Asking patients about the extent of their pain communicates empathy toward those individuals. Problems occur when healthcare professionals are presumptuous about how a patient should or should not feel.

5. Practitioners rely on a variety of continuing education and clinical experiences to guide them toward successful management of pain. Inherent in this process is the ability to adapt to and change specific patient complaints. This process is dynamic and continuous; each experience should develop better decision-making skills for the future. Healthcare professionals gain confidence with successful decisions, which ultimately benefits the patient.

II. UNDERSTANDING FEAR AND ANXIETY

A. Definitions

1. Anxiety: "A nonspecific feeling of apprehension, worry, uneasiness, or dread, the source of which may be vague or unknown. A normal, **rational** reaction when one's body, lifestyle, values, or loved ones are threatened."[5] Anxiety may be accompanied by restlessness, tension, tachycardia, and dyspnea.[16]

Box 3-1	WORDS TO DESCRIBE PAIN IN OTHER LANGUAGES

Word	Language
Aloum	Arabic
Tong	Chinese
Pain	English
Douleur	French
Schmerz	German
Ponai	Greek
Kú-av	Hebrew
Dardh	Indian
Itami	Japanese
Wicayazan	Lakota (Native American)
Bol	Polish
Bolit	Russian
Dolor	Spanish
Agn	Turkish
Dau	Vietnamese

2. Fear: "A feeling of fright or dread related to an identifiable source recognized by the individual."[5]
3. Phobia: "Any persistent and **irrational** fear of something specific, such as an object, activity, or situation that results in avoidance or desire to avoid the feared stimulus."[5] "Fear that is recognized as being excessive or unreasonable."[16]

B. Interaction between fear and pain

Fear and pain are so interrelated that they are often hard to separate. Both have physiologic and emotional components.[17] As pain increases, anxiety is heightened; as anxiety increases, pain becomes enhanced and, therefore, less tolerable.[6] In a medical setting, children cite fear of pain to be a significant obstacle.[18] When fear or pain is an issue, both must ultimately be managed.

C. Assessing and measuring fear and anxiety

1. Objectively quantifying a patient's fear or anxiety poses a dilemma similar to pain. There are several methods of assessing fear. Physiologic and behavioral signs often are overt indicators of fear ("white knuckle syndrome" is depicted in Figure 3-5). A simple interview with a patient will uncover otherwise unspoken concerns. Similar to scales used with pain, many measurement devices indicate fear and anxiety. The literature overflows with suggested indicators.[19-21] Although modified, a classic, five-item, anxiety questionnaire developed by Norman Corah asks patients to identify the level of anxiety associated with imminent dental treatment and specific procedures such as drilling, cleaning, and administration of a local anesthetic[22] (Box 3-2). In addition, crying, clinging, sweating, syncope, refusal to cooperate, and obsessive talking may be interpreted as signs of fear. Chronic tardiness or last-minute appointment cancellations may also possibly be anxiety related.
2. Repeatedly, we hear of patients carrying fear into their adult lives precipitated from a negative childhood experience in a medical or dental setting. Often patients have preconceived expectations of pain stemming from attitudes and behaviors displayed by parents, siblings, coworkers, significant others, etc.[18] For those patients who have significant fear or phobias, referral to an appropriate professional (i.e., child psychologist) is suggested. Many management options are available for these individuals.[23]

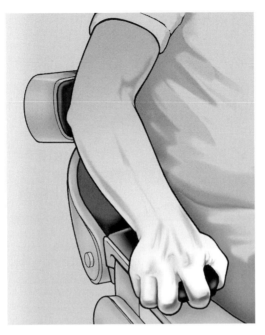

Figure 3-5 Fear can be visible.

Box 3-2 | **MODIFIED DENTAL ANXIETY SCALE (MDAS)**

1. If you went to your dentist for treatment tomorrow, how would you feel?
   Not Anxious   Slightly Anxious   Fairly Anxious   Very Anxious   Extremely Anxious

2. If you were sitting in the waiting room (waiting for treatment), how would you feel?
   Not Anxious   Slightly Anxious   Fairly Anxious   Very Anxious   Extremely Anxious

3. If you were about to have a tooth drilled, how would you feel?
   Not Anxious   Slightly Anxious   Fairly Anxious   Very Anxious   Extremely Anxious

4. If you were about to have your teeth scaled and polished, how would you feel?
   Not Anxious   Slightly Anxious   Fairly Anxious   Very Anxious   Extremely Anxious

5. If you were about to have a local anesthetic injection in your gum above your upper back tooth, how would you feel?
   Not Anxious   Slightly Anxious   Fairly Anxious   Very Anxious   Extremely Anxious

Total score is a sum of all five items, ranging from 5–25 (Not Anxious = 1; Extremely Anxious = 5). Nineteen or greater indicates a highly dentally anxious patient or possibly a dental phobic.

It is crucial that every effort be made to ensure a positive experience for each patient, child or adult.

D. Acknowledgment of fear and anxiety

   1. Good communication skills are necessary to facilitate the interpersonal interaction between the patient and provider. The basic fundamentals of good communication

include warmth, empathy, and respect.[24] Empathy, which is best expressed through eye contact, has been cited as the greatest attribute a healthcare professional can possess.[25] By disclosing a genuine caring attitude, kindness, and concern for patients, healthcare providers can facilitate an interaction that allows for effective problem solving.[24] Patients do not care what providers know until they know that they care.

2. Appropriate acknowledgment of patients' anxiety can solidify their confidence and allow an informed review of potential management options specific to every individual.[4]

III. SEDATION LEVELS AS DEFINED BY THE ASA PRACTICE GUIDELINES FOR SEDATION AND ANALGESIA BY NON-ANESTHESIOLOGISTS[26] (BOX 3-3)

A. **Definitions**

1. Minimal sedation (anxiolysis): a drug-induced state during which patients respond normally to verbal commands. Although cognitive function and coordination may be impaired, ventilatory and cardiovascular functions are unaffected. When administering N_2O, minimal sedation is accomplished when concentrations are less than 50%.

2. Moderate sedation-analgesia: a drug-induced depression of consciousness during which patients respond *purposefully*[27] to verbal commands, either alone or accompanied by light tactile stimulation. No interventions are required to maintain a patent airway, and spontaneous ventilation is adequate. Cardiovascular function is usually maintained. Moderate sedation is achieved when N_2O concentrations are greater than 50%. Reflex withdrawal from a painful stimulus is *not* considered a purposeful response.[27]

3. Deep sedation-analgesia: a drug-induced depression of consciousness during which patients cannot be easily aroused but respond *purposefully*[27] after repeated or painful stimulation. The ability to independently maintain ventilatory function may be impaired. Patients may require assistance in maintaining a patent airway, and spontaneous ventilation may be inadequate. Cardiovascular function is usually maintained. Reflex withdrawal from a painful stimulus is *not* considered a purposeful response.[27]

4. General anesthesia: a drug-induced loss of consciousness during which patients are not arousable, even by painful stimulation. The ability to independently maintain ventilatory function is often impaired. Patients often require assistance in maintaining a patent airway, and positive pressure ventilation may be required because of depressed spontaneous ventilation or drug-induced depression of neuromuscular function. Cardiovascular function may be impaired. With N_2O/O_2, it is difficult to reach the appropriate plane for performing a surgical procedure; however, although difficult, it is possible to render a patient unconscious with N_2O/O_2.

B. **Sedation as a continuum**

Because sedation is a continuum, it is not always possible to predict how an individual patient will respond. Hence, practitioners intending to produce a given level of sedation should be able to rescue patients whose level of sedation becomes deeper than initially intended. Individuals administering minimal sedation should be able to rescue patients who enter a state of

Box 3-3	ASA CONTINUUM OF DEPTH OF SEDATION	
	Minimal sedation (anxiolysis)	Deep sedation-analgesia
	Moderate sedation-analgesia	General anesthesia

moderate sedation; those administering moderate sedation-analgesia should be able to rescue patients who enter a state of deep sedation-analgesia, and those administering deep sedation-analgesia should be able to rescue patients who enter a state of general anesthesia.

IV. SPECTRUM OF PAIN AND ANXIETY MANAGEMENT OPTIONS

A. Several options are available for managing a patient's pain and anxiety. The spectrum begins with no intervention and ends with general anesthesia (Figure 3-6). There are methods that use pharmacologic agents and others that do not. Options for consideration will be discussed briefly. For additional information regarding any of these, several reputable texts and other resources are available.[3]

1. Noninvasive, nonpharmacologic approach to sedation
   a. Words and actions are used by a clinician to facilitate a trusting relationship and positive rapport with a patient. This conscious choice of verbal and nonverbal communication is a vital component of every patient–operator interaction.[28] Positive attitudes, welcoming smiles, and a genuine display of kindness and concern reassure patients and may be all that is necessary to allay fear and anxiety. Language and actions are calm, slow, relaxing, and gentle.[29] Often, word choice and tone are used to facilitate the effectiveness of pharmacologic modalities.
   b. Hypnosis is another nonpharmacologic method of providing pain and anxiety relief. Promoters suggest that hypnosis makes use of an individual's natural abilities.[30] Further study and training are necessary before the use of these techniques in addition to patient preparation. Annual courses are sponsored by the Society for Developmental and Behavioral Pediatrics.[15] Not everyone is hypnosuggestable; therefore, this option is not reliable for all patients.
   c. Acupuncture and acupressure are similar to hypnosis because they require further education and training before they are used.[15,31] Their disadvantage, similar to hypnosis, is unreliability for every patient.
   d. Systematic desensitization, relaxation therapy, biofeedback, and other coping strategies may be used to manage patient fear and anxiety.[15] These methods usually require the assistance of specialized professionals. Many resources are available that provide such services and/or information.
   e. Distraction mechanisms are intended to divert the individual's attention away from a fear-provoking stimulus. Examples of such distractions are reading materials in reception areas, music through office speakers or headphones, television, movies, aromatherapy, virtual reality headsets, sky and seascape scenes within ceiling lights, and even manicures during dental procedures (Figure 3-5).
   f. Transcutaneous electrical nerve stimulation (TENS) and electronic dental anesthesia (EDA) are pain-relieving methods that use electricity to prevent impulses from reaching the brain. Large A fibers are stimulated electrically until the patient signals a tolerable twitching sensation. According to the Melzack and Wall[32] gate theory, impulses will not be propagated further, thus reducing pain. TENS also acts with the endogenous opioid system to produce endorphins and enkephalins.[33] Historically, TENS has been used in physical therapy; however, dentistry has given TENS and EDA more exposure. The first and only blind controlled study of TENS effectiveness was done by Clark et al.[34] Several other studies indicate significant analgesic effects.[15,35–37]

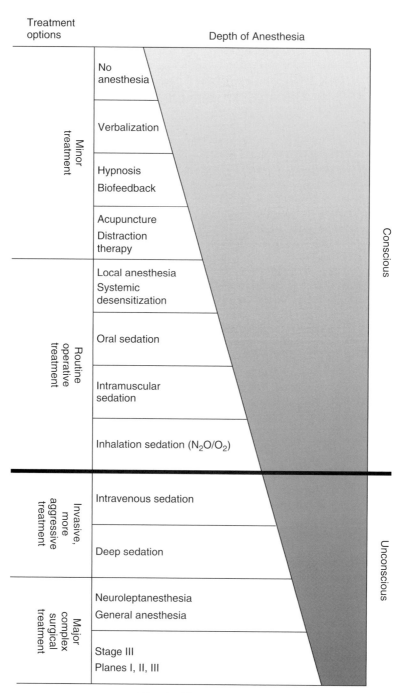

Figure 3-6 Pain and anxiety management options.

2. Invasive, pharmacologic approach to sedation
    a. Conscious patients
        i. Local anesthesia is described as a loss of sensation in a localized area caused by an anesthetic agent that blocks the neurotransmission of impulses to the brain. The injection is known to be a primary source of the fear and anxiety that providers continuously attempt to manage.[38] However, local anesthesia is the backbone for pain management, especially in dentistry.
        ii. The oral route may be used to administer pharmacologic agents for the purpose of relaxing an apprehensive individual without producing unconsciousness.[4] Administering drugs orally is universally accepted by the general population. Patient cooperation is necessary but usually not problematic, except with children in some cases. Oral medication has a latent period of 30 minutes, peaking at approximately 1 hour, and may be considerably affected by gastric contents. Duration of action and recovery are prolonged, and an escort is often required. This enteral sedation technique has become popular of late. However, it is fraught with potential complications when nitrous oxide is used in combination with oral drugs that are almost impossible to titrate. There is no mechanism for titration with oral medication.
        iii. The intramuscular (IM) route of administration is accomplished by direct injection into muscular tissue. Clinical action is more rapid than with the oral route, and absorption is more reliable. Disadvantages are the inability to titrate the drug, prolonged duration, incomplete recovery, and the necessity for an injection.[4]
        iv. The inhalation route of administration of medication offers many advantages and few disadvantages. The clinical effect is rapid, titration is possible, and elimination of the drug is usually rapid. This will be discussed as it pertains to N_2O in greater detail in Chapter 4.
        v. The IV route of administration is the direct deposition of drug into the circulatory system. This allows for very rapid response and onset of action. It is titratable and, therefore, can be tailored for a specific procedure. Recovery time can be prolonged, and the patient requires an escort.[4]
    b. Unconscious patients
        i. General anesthesia has been used extensively in the health professions since the discovery of ether as an anesthetic. Patient cooperation is not a factor for its effectiveness, which is often the reason why this modality is selected. Patients who are unmanageable for any reason are potential candidates for general anesthesia. To perform this technique, the practitioner must complete additional educational requirements and assume greater liability.[4]
B. Whichever option is chosen, careful and competent decision-making skills are vital. Select the management option that best suits the situation at hand. Because each person responds differently to pharmacologic and nonpharmacologic methods of treatment, remember that an individual's responses are variable on any given day. Psychological and physiologic factors must be considered at each meeting with the patient. When one approach is insufficient or undesirable, another may prove effective.

REFERENCES

1. American Pain Society: Press room, media backgrounder, *"Impact of untreated and undertreated pain"*, Accessed from *www.ampainsoc.org*, June 2006.
2. Consensus Conference: Anesthesia and sedation in the dental office, *J Am Med Assoc* 254:1073, 1985.
3. Sprouls LS: Dealing with dental phobics, *Dent Team* 5(6):14, 1992.
4. Malamed SF: *Sedation: A Guide to Patient Management*, ed 4, St. Louis, 2003, Mosby.
5. Thomas CL, ed: *Taber's Cyclopedic Medical Dictionary*, Philadelphia, 1997, FA Davis.
6. Stoelting RK: *Pharmacology and Physiology in Anesthetic Practice*, ed 2, Philadelphia, 1991, JB Lippincott.
7. Hirst M: The changing nature of pain control: clinical aspects of endorphins and enkephalins, *J Can Dent Assoc* 51:493, 1985.
8. Gillman MA: Analgesic (subanesthetic) nitrous oxide interacts with the endogenous opioid system: a review of the evidence, *Life Sciences* 39:1209, 1986.
9. Reisine T, Pasternak G: Opioid analgesics and antagonists. In Hardman JG, Limbird LE, editors: *Goodman and Gillman's: the Pharmacologic Basis of Therapeutics*, ed 9, New York, 1996, McGraw-Hill.
10. Hargreaves KM, Milam SB: Mechanisms of orofacial pain and analgesia. In Dionne RA, Phero JC, Becker DE, editors: *Management of Pain and Anxiety in the Dental Office*, St. Louis, 2002, Saunders.
11. American Academy of Pediatrics and American Pain Society: The assessment and management of acute pain in infants, children, and adolescents, *Pediatrics* 108(3):793, 2001.
12. Kohr J: Measuring your patient's pain, *RN* 58:39, 1995.
13. Gujol MC: A survey of pain assessment and management practices among critical care nurses, *Am J Crit Care* 3:123, 1994.
14. McCafery M, Richey KJ: Techniques of pain assessment, *Nurse Week* 5:16, 1992.
15. Zempsky WT, Schechter NL: What's new in the management of pain in children, *Pediatr Rev* 24:337, 2003.
16. *Dorland's Illustrated Medical Dictionary*, ed 31, Philadelphia, 2007, Elsevier.
17. Dionne RA, Kaneko Y: Overcoming pain and anxiety in dentistry. In Dionne RA, Phero JC, Becker DE, editors: *Management of Pain and Anxiety in Dental Practice*, St. Louis, 2002, Saunders.
18. Prins PJ: Anxiety in medical settings. In Ollendick TH, King NJ, Yule W, editors: *International Handbook of Phobic and Anxiety Disorders in Children and Adolescents*, New York, 1994, Plenum Press.
19. Mendola P, O'Shea RM, Zielezny MA: Validity and reliability of the interval scale of anxiety response, *Anesth Prog* 34:202, 1987.
20. Parkin SF: The assessment of two dental anxiety rating scales for children, *J Dent Child* 55:269, 1988.
21. Elter JR, Strauss RP, Beck JD: Assessing dental anxiety, dental care use and oral status in older adults, *J Am Dent Assoc* 128:591, 1997.
22. Newton JT, Edwards JC: Psychometric properties of the modified dental anxiety scale: an independent replication, *Community Dental Health* 22(1):40, 2005.
23. Weinstein P, Nathan JE: The challenge of fearful and phobic children, *Dent Clin North Am* 32:667, 1988.
24. Doebling S, Rowe MM: Negative perceptions of dental stimuli and their effects on dental fear, *J Dent Hygiene* 74:110, 2000.
25. Ketchum C: Freedom from fear, *RDH* 3:14, 1995.
26. ASA Task Force: Practice guidelines for sedation and analgesia by non-anesthesiologists, *Anesthesiology* 96(4):1007, 2002.
27. AAP/AAPD Clinical Report: Guidelines for monitoring and management of pediatric patients during and after sedation for diagnostic and therapeutic procedures: an update, *Pediatrics* 118(6):2587, December 2006.
28. Stracher K: The role of suggestion in conscious-sedation, *Anesth Prog* 23:59, 1976.
29. Ross ID: Fear control with nitrous oxide sedation, *SAAD Digest* 9:69, 1992.
30. Simpson MA, *et al: Hypnosis in Dentistry: A Handbook for Clinical Use*, Springfield, Ill, 1985, Charles C Thomas.
31. Santamaria LB: Non-pharmacologic techniques for treatment of post-operative pain, *Minerva Anesthesiol* 56:359, 1990.
32. Melzack R, Wall P: Pain mechanisms: a new theory, *Science* 150:971, 1965.
33. Malamed SF: *Handbook of Local Anesthesia*, ed 5, St. Louis, 2004, Mosby.
34. Clark MS *et al:* An evaluation of the clinical analgesia/anesthesia efficacy on acute pain using the high frequency neural modulator in various dental settings, *Oral Surg* 63:501, 1987.

35. Christensen GJ: Electronic anesthesia: research and thoughts, *J Calif Dent Assoc* 15:46, 1987.
36. Hochman R: Neurotransmitter modulator (TENS) for control of dental operative pain, *J Am Dent Assoc* 116:208, 1988.
37. Malamed SF *et al*: Electronic dental anesthesia for restorative dentistry, *Anesth Prog* 36:195, 1989.
38. Milgrom P *et al*: Four dimensions of fear of dental injections, *J Am Dent Assoc* 128:756, 1997.

SUGGESTED READINGS

Heitkemper T, Layne C, Sullivan DM: Brief treatment of children's dental pain and anxiety, *Percept Mot Skills* 76:192, 1993.
Kaufman E, Jastak JT: Sedation for outpatient dental procedures, *Compend Dent* 16:462, 1995.
Nathan JE: Management of the difficult child: a survey of pediatric dentists' use of restraints, sedation and general anesthesia, *J Dent Child* 56(4):293, 1989.
Slavin HC: What we know about pain, *J Am Dent Assoc* 127:1536, 1996.

Desirable Characteristics of N_2O/O_2 Sedation

N_2O/O_2 sedation has many advantages over other pain and anxiety management options. Many indications exist for its use, and the disadvantages are few; for these reasons it can be a useful sedative method. Most of these advantages deal with the pharmacokinetics of the drug itself (Box 4-1). Judge for yourself how the N_2O/O_2 option compares with others.

I. DESIRABLE CHARACTERISTICS OF N_2O/O_2 SEDATION

A. Analgesic properties (pain control)

1. Chapman et al[1] state that a mixture of 20% N_2O and 80% O_2 has the same analgesic equipotence as 15 mg of morphine. Other methods verifying the analgesic efficacy of N_2O have been reported.[2]
2. The level of pain control afforded by N_2O can vary from patient to patient because of individual biovariability; however, the analgesic properties of N_2O are well recognized and its potency is significant.[1] These analgesic properties are useful even with the severe pain associated with myocardial infarction.[3] N_2O has the ability to raise the patient's pain threshold when administered before intraoral injections in dentistry.[4]
3. N_2O/O_2 is also advantageous when other analgesic drugs are contraindicated (i.e., allergy).
4. Fear affects an individual's ability to tolerate pain; painful stimuli can be exaggerated in an anxious patient. A common fear is fear of an injection or a needle (i.e., vaccination), which can intensify an individual's reaction to pain.[5] N_2O has the ability to manage both pain and fear.

B. Anxiolytic properties (sedative effects)

1. Patient anxiety has long been associated with healthcare.[6] A person's mental ability to cope with certain situations can depend on such things as age, gender, previous experiences, and personality characteristics.[7]
2. N_2O/O_2 therapy can significantly assist patients in handling their fear or anxiety by producing sedation or a sense of well-being. Sedation enables the patient to become calm, relaxed, and able to tolerate the situation better or with no difficulty. Jackson and Johnson concur that N_2O/O_2 sedation is an "excellent choice" for managing mild fear.[8]
   a. This relaxed feeling has a positive effect on the patient's pain threshold.
   b. Mood changes with N_2O have been studied. Zacny et al[9] report positive mood changes in patients with high anxiety and in those with low anxiety. Children older than 6 were less distressed during nitrous oxide administration as reported by Kanagasundaram et al.[10]

Box 4-1	DESIRABLE CHARACTERISTICS OF N_2O

Analgesic   Titration possible
Anxiolytic   Rapid and complete recovery
Relative amnestic   Minimal side effects
Rapid onset of action

   c. Patients with dental fear were treated with N_2O/O_2 sedation. Results were favorable; studies reassessed patients 1 and 5 years later. The results showed that the N_2O treatment method still had a positive effect.[11,12]
   3. In treatment of pediatric patients, N_2O/O_2 has been shown to facilitate positive behavior and lowered anxiety levels on sequential visits.[13] It is a continuing goal of all healthcare providers to prevent negative early childhood experiences to reduce the number of fearful adults. Ultimately, the goal is to provide patients with enough positive experiences that they do not require N_2O/O_2 sedation in the future.

C. Amnestic properties
   1. The amnestic property of N_2O/O_2 sedation is another of its positive attributes.[14] Postoperatively, patients often state they cannot recall the severity of their pain or anxiety or its duration.
   2. The passage of time tends to become unclear or compressed under N_2O/O_2 sedation. A patient may remark how quickly time passed during a long procedure.[4]

D. Onset of action
   1. N_2O/O_2 sedation has a rapid onset of action. Because of the pharmacologic characteristics of N_2O, clinical effects may begin in less than 30 seconds, with peak effects usually occurring in less than 5 minutes.
   2. Another conscious-sedative modality that closely parallels the rapid onset of clinical action of N_2O/O_2 is IV sedation.

E. Titration
   1. Titration is the process of administering a drug incrementally to a specific level or endpoint of sedation. It allows for the exact amount of the drug necessary to be delivered to every patient at every appointment. Titration is very easily accomplished with N_2O/O_2 sedation. N_2O is one of several drugs that accommodate the concept of titration well.
   2. Titration is also possible with IV sedation; however, in this case, reversal is not as straightforward as with N_2O.

F. Recovery
   1. Inhalation of N_2O/O_2 allows for complete recovery with 100% pure oxygen for a minimum of 5 minutes after termination of the drug. Depending on patient assessment, individual recovery time may vary. Recovery will be discussed further in Chapter 14.

G. Elimination
   1. Nitrous oxide is 99% eliminated from the body within 5–10 minutes after discontinuation of use. Therefore, at the conclusion of recovery, cognitive function is not affected.[4]

H. Acceptance

1. Patient acceptance of the procedure has been well documented. Berge[15] states that the acceptance rate is the same for oral surgery procedures as it is for general dentistry.

II. COMBINING N_2O/O_2 SEDATION WITH OTHER METHODS

A. N_2O/O_2 sedation is enhanced with the spoken word. Soothing, calm, humorous, encouraging words and actions of the operator facilitate the relaxing effects of the drug.[4,16] Investigators believe the psychologic preparation of the patient before N_2O/O_2 administration has a significant impact on its effects.[17-19]

B. Weinstein and Nathan[20] indicate that N_2O used in combination with distraction techniques was more effective than distraction with a placebo gas when working with children. They also suggest that the combination of N_2O/O_2 and hypnosis and imagery was effective with their population.[20]

C. Another combination cited as effective with pediatric patients is the use of audio-analgesia and N_2O/O_2. The addition of music as an adjuvant to N_2O/O_2 sedation was positive for the children studied (Figure 4-1).[21] Music has been used as a method for calming, relaxing, and distracting individuals in the healthcare setting since the era of unusually loud music used for distraction (also known as "white sound") in the late 1950s and early 1960s.[22,23]

D. An interesting development by a Boston-area anesthesiologist has entered the market and is designed to assist nitrous oxide/oxygen sedation procedures with young children. His experience as an emergency room physician led him to design a snorkel-like headset that delivers nitrous oxide and oxygen while simultaneously allowing the child to listen to music or play with a Nintendo GameBoy.[24] In addition, this device monitors the child's respiration and oxygen saturation levels (Figure 4-2).

E. Quarnstrom[25] was more successful in his research when he combined N_2O/O_2 and EDA, compared with the use of each modality alone. Donaldson et al[26] had similar results.

F. Oral premedication may be used safely with N_2O/O_2 sedation.[27] Diazepam and meperidine have been cited as drugs used concomitantly with N_2O. However, several other drugs and delivery methods have been used with nitrous oxide.[28-30] Although the effects of

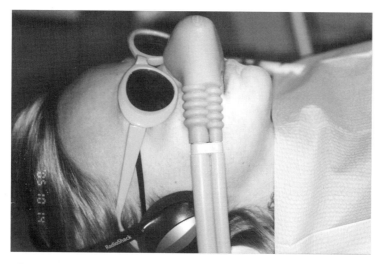

Figure 4-1 Music and N_2O/O_2 sedation. *(Courtesy of Dr. Elizabeth Barr, Denver, Colorado.)*

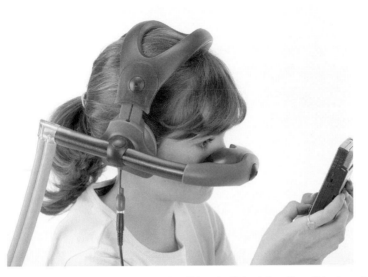

Figure 4-2 PediSedate delivers N_2O/O_2 sedation while allowing the child to play Nintendo GameBoy or listen to music. *(Courtesy of Design Continuum.)*

nitrous oxide are easily reversed with oxygen, practitioners must be responsible and accountable for all other drugs administered to their patients and the potential adverse situations that could ensue.

G. The combination that deserves special attention is that of N_2O/O_2 and local anesthesia. The benefits of local anesthesia are apparent; N_2O/O_2 should not be used as a substitute for local anesthesia but rather in combination with it. If N_2O/O_2 is administered alone in a situation that also requires local anesthesia, the patient may blame the N_2O/O_2 unfairly for not eliminating the pain. The patient will be less likely to trust N_2O/O_2 in the future. Local anesthesia and N_2O/O_2 combined offer a superior pain and anxiety management option.[15]

REFERENCES

1. Chapman WP, Arrowood JG, Beecher HK: The analgesic effects of low concentrations of nitrous oxide compared in man with morphine sulphate, *J Clin Invest* 22:871, 1943.
2. Pirec V, Patterson TH, Thapar P: Effects of subanesthetic concentrations of nitrous oxide on cold-pressor pain in humans, *Pharm Biochem Behav* 51:323, 1995.
3. Thompson PL, Lown B: Nitrous oxide as an analgesic in acute myocardial infarction, *JAMA* 235:924, 1976.
4. Malamed SF: *Sedation: A Guide to Patient Management,* ed 4, St Louis, 2003, Mosby.
5. Murray JB: Psychology of the pain experience. In Weisenberg M, editor: *Pain: Clinical and Experimental Perspectives,* St Louis, 1975, Mosby.
6. Doebling S, Rowe MM: Negative perceptions of dental stimuli and their effects on dental fear, *JDH* 74(II):110, 2000.
7. Doerr PA *et al*: Factors associated with dental anxiety, *J Am Dent Assoc* 129:1111, 1998.
8. Jackson DL, Johnson BS: Inhalational and enteral conscious sedation for the adult dental patient, *Dent Clin North Am* 46(4):781, 2002.
9. Zacny JP *et al*: Preoperative dental anxiety and mood changes during nitrous oxide inhalation, *J Am Dent Assoc* 133:82, 2002.
10. Kanagasundaram SA *et al*: Efficacy and safety of nitrous oxide in alleviating pain and anxiety during painful procedures, *Arch Dis Child* 84:492, 2001.

11. Willumsen T et al: One-year follow-up of patients treated for dental fear: effects of cognitive therapy, applied relaxations, and nitrous oxide sedation, *Acta Odontol Scand* 59(6):335, 2001.
12. Willumsen T, Vassend O: Effects of cognitive therapy, applied relaxation and nitrous oxide sedation. A five-year follow-up study of patients treated for dental fear, *Acta Odont Scand* 61(2):93, 2003.
13. Veerkamp JS et al: Anxiety reduction with nitrous oxide: a permanent solution? *J Dent Child* 62:44, 1995.
14. Ramsey DS, Leonesio RJ, Whitney CW et al: Paradoxical effects of nitrous oxide on human memory, *Psychopharmacology* 106:370, 1992.
15. Berge TI: Acceptance and side effects of nitrous oxide oxygen sedation for oral surgical procedures, *Acta Odontol Scand* 57(4):201, 1999.
16. Winland RD: Humor: part of the treatment plan, *Gen Dentistry* 45(5):414, 1997.
17. Patel B et al: The use of hypnosis in dentistry: a review, *Dent Update* 27(4):198, 2002.
18. Dworkin SF et al: Analgesic effects of nitrous oxide with controlled painful stimuli, *J Am Dent Assoc* 107:581, 1983.
19. Chaves JF: Recent advances in the application of hypnosis to pain management, *Am J Clin Hypn* 37:117, 1994.
20. Weinstein P, Nathan JE: The challenge of fearful and phobic children, *Dent Clin North Am* 32:667, 1988.
21. Anderson WD: The effectiveness of audio-nitrous oxide-oxygen psychosedation on dental behavior of a child, *J Pedodontics* 5:3, 1980.
22. Gardner, Licklider: Auditory analgesia in dental operation, *J Am Dent Assoc* 59:1144, 1959.
23. Robson, Davenport: The effects of white sound and music upon superficial pain threshold, *Can J Anaesth* 9:105, 1962.
24. Denman WT et al: The PediSedate device, a novel approach to pediatric sedation that provides distraction and inhaled nitrous oxide: clinical evaluation in a large case series, *Pediatr Anesth* 17(2):162, 2007.
25. Quarnstrom FC: Clinical experience with TENS and TENS combined with nitrous oxide-oxygen, *Anesth Prog* 36:66, 1989.
26. Donaldson D, Quarnstrom F, Jastak JT: The combined effect of nitrous oxide and oxygen and electrical stimulation during restorative dental treatment, *J Am Dent Assoc* 118(6):733, 1989.
27. Jastak JT, Paravecchio R: An analysis of 1331 sedations using inhalation, intravenous, or other techniques, *J Am Dent Assoc* 91:1242, 1975.
28. Lahoud GY, Averley PA: Comparison of sevoflurane and nitrous oxide mixture with nitrous oxide alone for inhalation conscious sedation in children having dental treatment: a randomised controlled trial, *Anaesthesia* 57:446, 2002.
29. Averley PA et al: A randomised controlled trial of paediatric conscious sedation for dental treatment using intravenous midazolam combines with inhaled nitrous oxide or nitrous oxide/sevoflurane, *Anaesthesia* 59:844, 2004.
30. Gries DA et al: Anxiolytic-like action in mice treated with nitrous oxide and oral triazolam or diazepam, *Life Sciences* 76:1667, 2005.

Physical Properties and Pharmacokinetics/ Pharmacodynamics of N_2O

T he conscientious healthcare provider offering N_2O/O_2 sedation to patients must be knowledgeable about the physical properties, as well as the pharmacokinetics and pharmacodynamics of any drug they administer. Pharmacokinetics is defined as "the activity or fate of drugs in the body over a period of time, including the processes of absorption, distribution, localization in tissues, biotransformation, and excretion."[1] The definition of pharmacodynamics is "the study of the biochemical and physiological effects of drugs and the mechanisms of their actions, including the correlation of actions and effects of drugs with their chemical structure, and the effects on the actions of a drug or drugs."[1] N_2O has many favorable attributes, which prove noteworthy in the ambulatory setting. After having reviewed the attributes of nitrous oxide in the previous chapter, its usefulness is apparent. Although there may be disagreement about whether N_2O deserves the "ideal" label, many agree that its role in healthcare is fundamental.

I. PHYSICAL AND CHEMICAL PROPERTIES OF N_2O

A. Dinitrogen monoxide (N_2O) is a stable, linear compound that is chemically diagrammed as $N \equiv N = O$. It is a sweet-smelling, colorless gas.
B. The boiling point of N_2O, which is 88.5° C (127° F), indicates that it is a gas at room temperature. When compressed into a cylinder, N_2O becomes a liquid.
C. The substance itself is nonflammable; however, N_2O supports combustion. If the gas comes in contact with a combustible substance or flame, decomposition of the gas will occur. If the decomposition occurs at high temperature and elevated pressure (inside a cylinder or high-pressure pipeline), a violent chemical reaction such as an explosion will occur. If N_2O is present near an open flame, the flame will burn brighter.[2]
D. Because N_2O like O_2 is an oxidizing gas, no hydrocarbon compounds, such as lubricants, grease, or oil, should be used on any N_2O storage, distribution, or dispensing equipment. Of further concern is the operation of such equipment in a manner that increases the temperature of the N_2O. The most common example is the quick opening of valves, which causes a rapid pressure increase. The phenomenon known as the heat of compression can increase the temperature of the metal to a level that ignites any hydrocarbon contaminants and causes a chemical reaction resulting in fire or explosion. This reaction can occur with any organic contaminant acting as a fuel.
E. The molecular weight of N_2O is 44. Its specific gravity is 1.53, which indicates that it is heavier than air (gr = 1) or pure O_2 (gr = 1.1).
F. N_2O is found in minimal concentrations (319 ppb) in the atmosphere.[3]

Anesthetic N_2O contributes insignificantly to that total amount.[3] As ultraviolet (UV) light combines with N_2O and O_2, free radicals (i.e., nitric oxide) are produced, which can affect the ozone.[4] Several natural and man-made methods release N_2O into the atmosphere (e.g., burning of pine wood). The US Environmental Protection Agency (EPA) and others suggest that N_2O enters the environment through rivers and ocean currents, denitrification of soil, through livestock manure and human sewage, as well as plants and trees.[3–7] Concentrations of this naturally occurring greenhouse gas have increased 18% from 1750, a preindustrial time period, to 2004, whereas carbon dioxide (CO_2) and methane (NH_4) have increased 35% and 143%, respectively.[3]

II. PHYSICAL AND CHEMICAL PROPERTIES OF O_2

A. Discovery

1. Many early scientists, such as Bayen, Borch, and Scheele, prepared O_2 but did not recognize the significance of their findings.[8]
2. Joseph Priestley in England was credited with discovering not only N_2O but also O_2, carbon monoxide, sulfur dioxide, and ammonia. Priestley, a British chemist, is considered one of the founders of modern chemistry because of his contributions to the field of science.[9]

B. Preparation

1. O_2 is primarily prepared by fractional evaporation of liquid air or by heating potassium chlorate by use of manganese dioxide as a catalyst. Air separation manufacturing facilities make 99% of the gas. O_2 costs approximately 5 cents per cubic foot for small quantities.[8]
2. Air is cooled and compressed until it liquefies. O_2 compresses to a pale blue liquid at $-183°$ C.
3. Nitrogen (N) and other elements evaporate, leaving liquid O_2.
4. Oxygen is also produced by plants during photosynthesis.

C. Characteristics

1. In a gaseous state, O_2 is odorless, colorless, and tasteless.
2. It makes up approximately 21% of the earth's atmosphere and makes up 49.2% of the earth's crust. The human body is 61% oxygen and 90% of water is oxygen. Oxygen is the third most abundant element in the sun and is thought to be part of its energy source.[8]
3. The molecular weight of O_2 is 32; its specific gravity is 1.1 (air = 1), and its atomic weight is 15.9. The atomic weight of oxygen was used as the standard for comparison of other elements until carbon 12 replaced it as the standard in 1961.[8]
4. Like N_2O, O_2 supports combustion but is not itself flammable. It reacts similarly to N_2O when it contacts a combustible material such as oils, grease, or flammable materials.
5. O_2 is a compressed gas in cylinders. The dial in the regulator gauge accurately depicts the O_2 content in the cylinder. As the gas is consumed, the dial changes proportionally.
6. Oxygen is highly reactive and combines with most elements. It is a component within hundreds of thousands of organic compounds.

D. Uses

1. There are many uses for O_2. The steel industry is one of the largest consumers of O_2. O_2 is also used for welding and lighting and as a propellant in rockets. It is widely used in the medical field for surgical procedures, treating anaerobic infections, and hypoxia. Commercially, O_2 consumption is estimated at 20 million short tons per year in the United States.[8]

2. O_2 is the required component of N_2O when N_2O is used for sedation. Current sedation equipment described guarantees a minimum O_2 delivery of 30%. This provides an amount of O_2 greater than that found naturally in atmospheric air, which is significant for patient safety during N_2O/O_2 administration. It is common to use approximately 2.5 tanks of O_2 to every 1 tank of N_2O during sedation procedures.

3. The oxygen molecule does not separate from the nitrogen molecule in N_2O and is therefore unavailable as an oxygen source.

III. PHARMACOKINETIC PROPERTIES OF N₂O

A. The pharmacokinetic aspects of a drug affect its uptake, distribution, metabolism, and elimination in the body. Inhaled agents such as N_2O express their actions on the body by moving across partial pressure gradients. The agent moves from a higher- to a lower-pressure gradient. Uptake, distribution, onset of action, and ultimately, recovery from anesthesia or sedation depend on the solubility and potency of the drug. The interaction between a drug, the brain, and other tissues until equilibrium is reached is expressed in values called partition coefficients. These values indicate the ease or difficulty of drug transfer to the brain and body.

1. The difference between the partial pressures of a gas (N_2O) and a liquid (blood) indicates how quickly the agent crosses the pulmonary membrane and enters the bloodstream. This is called the blood–gas partition coefficient. N_2O crosses the alveolar membrane easily. The solubility of the drug then determines how quickly equilibration occurs, and clinical action begins.

   a. If a drug is highly soluble, it will diffuse immediately into the blood and be distributed throughout the body. Its blood–gas partition coefficient will be high, indicating that more drug and/or more time will be necessary to achieve equilibration or the level necessary for movement of the agent to the brain.

   b. If a drug is relatively insoluble, equilibrium will be achieved quickly. The blood–brain barrier will be crossed rapidly, allowing the drug to reach the brain. The onset of clinical action will then also be rapid.

   c. N_2O is an example of a relatively insoluble drug. Its blood–gas partition coefficient is 0.47. It remains unchanged in the blood and does not combine with any blood elements; the O_2 component is not available for use in the body because N_2O does not break down. Uptake by the body is limited, indicating that equilibrium is achieved quickly. Therefore, peak clinical effects may be seen within 3–5 minutes after initiation of the agent.

   d. There is a major difference in partial pressure gradients between N_2O and nitrogen(N_2)(air). The partial pressure of N_2O is approximately 31 times greater than that of N_2 (Figure 5-1). Because of this, N_2O rapidly replaces the N_2 occupying any body space. Not only does N_2O physically replace N_2, but it also increases the volume and/or pressure of that space, depending on its rigid or nonrigid confines. Specific conditions regarding this phenomenon are described in Chapter 9 (Figure 5-2).

2. Other partition coefficients of N_2O between tissues, muscles, and fat are low. Equilibration occurs quickly in these instances because of the inability of the tissues to hold N_2O. Because of this, N_2O is not stored in the body to any extent; thus elimination is not impeded.[10]

B. Eger[11] introduced the concept of the concentration effect (Figure 5-3) of N_2O on induction. The concentration effect occurs when high concentrations of N_2O are delivered to

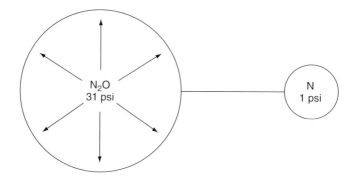

Figure 5-1 Partial pressure of N_2O is 31 times that of nitrogen (N_2).

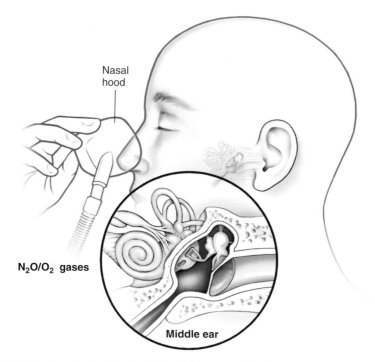

Figure 5-2 N_2O will diffuse from the blood into closed air-containing spaces in the body, like the middle ear, because it is 31 times more soluble than nitrogen. N_2O will continue to move into the space until equilibrium is achieved with the alveolar N_2O concentration. The higher the concentration of inspired N_2O, the more N_2O accumulates in the occluded middle ear, resulting in increased middle ear pressure because of the rigid confine.

the patient (70% N_2O). These high concentrations are often delivered during general anesthesia.

1. At high concentrations, alveolar partial pressures are reached rapidly, and there is little decrease in the concentration of the gas. In addition, when delivering these high concentrations of N_2O, the volume of inspired gas is increased. Negative pressure is produced, drawing more gas into the lungs and increasing the volume.

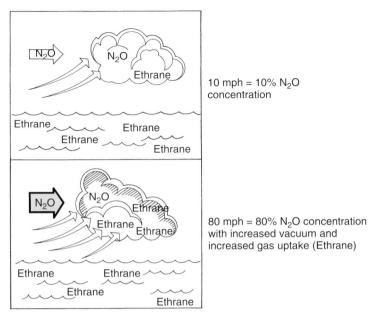

10 mph = 10% N_2O concentration

80 mph = 80% N_2O concentration with increased vacuum and increased gas uptake (Ethrane)

Figure 5-3 Concentration effect of N_2O.

2. At lower concentrations, the concentration effect is not significant. When administering analgesic percentages of N_2O, the rate of uptake is not as important.
C. Because high concentrations of N_2O promote the rapid uptake of the gas, there is a simultaneous effect occurring with the other gases being administered. The rapid uptake of N_2O allows the second gas to be drawn in much faster than it would normally if it were being administered alone. This phenomenon, called the "second-gas effect" (Figure 5-4), allows minimal amounts of a more potent anesthetic to be administered simultaneously with N_2O.[11]
D. N_2O is not metabolized through the liver. Ninety-nine percent of it is eliminated through the lungs without biotransformation.[12] A miniscule (0.004%) amount of N_2O is metabolized in the gastrointestinal tract. Reduction occurs by the anaerobic bacteria *Pseudomonas* and produces potentially toxic free radicals.[13,14] This process does not pose any significant threat to the body systems.
E. N_2O is difficult to use at extreme altitudes (i.e., above 10,000 feet). Because of the barometric pressure change, air ambulances and those administering N_2O/O_2 sedation at significant elevations must be aware of the need for an increase in N_2O concentration to obtain the same effects as at sea level.[12] In Denver, Colorado (5280 feet elevation), for example, a 5% increase in N_2O may be necessary compared with a location at sea level.

IV. PHARMACODYNAMICS OF NITROUS OXIDE

Pharmacodynamics is the study of the biochemical and physiologic effects of drugs and the mechanisms of their actions to include the correlation of those actions and effects of drugs with their chemical structure.[1] Knowledge of the mechanism in which nitrous oxide acts on the molecular level is limited; however, research is ongoing to determine its interaction with

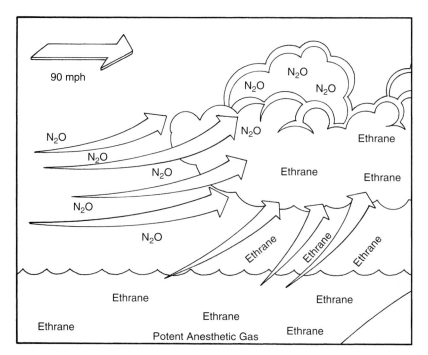

Figure 5-4 "Second-gas effect" associated with N_2O.

other inhalation agents commonly used in conjunction with it.[15–17] Therefore, the entirety of the pharmacodynamics of nitrous oxide is yet to be determined.

A. The potency of an anesthetic agent indicates how strong or powerful the drug is or how effective it is at producing anesthesia. There are many drugs available for general anesthesia that vary widely in potency.

   1. N_2O is the least potent (weakest) of all inhalation general anesthetics.

   2. Drug potency is determined by assessing the minimum alveolar concentration (MAC). MAC is defined as the amount of drug necessary to prevent movement in 50% of subjects responding to surgical incision.[18]

   3. The MAC for N_2O is 104%–105%. This value indicates that at normal atmospheric pressure, N_2O alone is not able to produce profound surgical anesthesia. N_2O can be used as the sole anesthetic agent under hyperbaric conditions.[19]

   4. The MAC value and limited potency of N_2O add tremendously to its safety. Some anesthetic agents and their corresponding MAC values are listed in Box 5-1.

B. Halothane, isoflurane, enflurane, desflurane, and sevoflurane are examples of more potent inhalation agents used for general anesthesia. Although their benefits are many, they also possess several negative factors, including toxicity, biotransformation, solubility, and general complication issues sometimes resulting in negative effects on organ systems.

C. N_2O can be used in combination with more potent inhaled agents to decrease the percentage of inhaled agents required and possibly diminish unwanted toxic side effects, as well as to be more cost-effective. The second-gas effect does not play a role per se in this regard. The second-gas effect is primarily relevant when trying to achieve equilibrium of the potent anesthetic agent, such as at induction.

Box 5-1	MINIMUM ALVEOLAR CONCENTRATION (MAC) VALUES FOR INHALATION ANESTHETICS	
	Anesthetic	**MAC Value**
	Desflurane	4.6%
	Enflurane	1.6%
	Halothane	0.75%
	Isoflurane	1.2%
	Nitrous oxide	104.0%
	Sevoflurane	1.7%

REFERENCES

1. Dorland NW: *Dorland's Illustrated Medical Dictionary*, ed 31, Philadelphia, 2007, Elsevier.
2. Fettes WC: Personal communication, August 1996.
3. United States Environmental Protection Agency: US greenhouse gas inventory report 1990–2004, http://epa.gov.
4. Dale O, Husum B: Nitrous oxide: a threat to personnel and global environment? *Acta Anaesthesiol Scand* 38:777, 1994.
5. Cole JJ, Caraco NF: Emissions of nitrous oxide from a tidal, freshwater river, the Hudson River, New York, *Environ Sci Technol* 35(6):991, 2001.
6. Barton L, Schipper LA: Regulation of nitrous oxide emissions from soils irrigated with dairy farm effluent, *J Environ Quality* 30(6):1881, 2001.
7. Xu H *et al*: N$_2$O emission by trees under natural conditions, *Environ Sci* 22(5):7, 2001.
8. Lide DR: *CRC Handbook of Chemistry and Physics*, ed 81, New York, 2001, CRC Press.
9. Microsoft Encarta Online Encyclopedia: Joseph Priestley, http://encarta.msn.com, 2002.
10. Eger EI II: Pharmacokinetics. In Eger EI II, editor: *Nitrous Oxide N$_2$O*, New York, 1985, Elsevier Science Publishing.
11. Eger EI II: Uptake and distribution. In Miller RD, editor: *Anesthesia*, ed 4, vol 1. New York, 1994, Churchill Livingstone.
12. Stoelting RD: *Pharmacology and Physiology in Anesthetic Practice*, ed 2, Philadelphia, 1991, JB Lippincott.
13. Hong K *et al*: Metabolism of nitrous oxide by human and rat intestinal contents, *Anesthesiology* 52:16, 1980.
14. Hong K *et al*: Biotransformation of nitrous oxide, *Anesthesiology* 53:354, 1980.
15. Woloszczuk-Gebicka B *et al*: Pharmacokinetic-pharmacodynamic relationship of rocuronium under stable nitrous oxide-fentanyl or nitrous oxide-sevoflurane anesthesia in children, *Paediatr Anaesth* 16(7):761, 2006.
16. Ropcke H *et al*: Isoflurane, nitrous oxide, and fentanyl pharmacodynamic interactions in surgical patients as measured by effects on median power frequency, *J Clin Anesth* 11(7):555, 1999.
17. Kansanaho M *et al*: dose-response and concentration-response relation of rocuronium infusion during propofol-nitrous oxide and isoflurane-nitrous oxide anaesthesia, *Eur J Anaesthesiol* 14(5):488, 1997.
18. Eger EI II, Saidman, LJ, Brandstater B: Minimum alveolar anesthetic concentration: a standard of anesthetic potency, *Anesthesiology* 26:756, 1965.
19. Eger EI II: MAC, In Eger EI II, editor: *Nitrous Oxide N$_2$O*, New York, 1985, Elsevier Science Publishing.

SUGGESTED READINGS

Cullen DJ: Anesthetic pharmacology and critical care, *Acute Care* 14–15:3, 1988–1989.
Dale O, Brown JR Jr: Clinical pharmacokinetics of the inhalational anaesthetics, *Clin Pharmacokinet* 12:145, 1987.
Hardman JG, Limbird LE, editors: *Goodman and Gillman's: The Pharmacologic Basis of Therapeutics*, ed 9, New York, 1996, McGraw-Hill.
Joyce JL: Inhalation anesthetics, *AORN J* 52:77, 1990.
Longnecker DE, Miller FL: Pharmacology of inhalation anesthetics. In Rogers M *et al*, editors: *Principles and Practice of Anesthesiology*, St Louis, 1993, Mosby.
Stenqvist O: Nitrous oxide kinetics, *Acta Anaesthesiol Scand* 38:757, 1994.

Manufacturing and Distribution of N_2O and O_2 Gases

I. MANUFACTURING

A. Process and storage

1. The manufacturing process for N_2O is relatively simple. The raw ingredient, ammonium nitrate (NH_4NO_3), is supplied as a clear liquid or as solid, pellet-sized particles. This material is used for fertilizer and as a primary ingredient of explosives.

2. To make N_2O, NH_4NO_3 is heated to approximately 250° C. At that point the NH_4NO_3 decomposes into N_2O, water (steam), and some contaminants ($NH_4NO_3 \rightarrow N_2O + 2\ H_2O$). The gas mixture is cooled to ambient room temperature, the steam is condensed, and most of the water is removed. The resulting crude N_2O gas mixture is scrubbed to extract the contaminants. The gas is then compressed, dried to remove the remaining water, cooled, and liquefied. The resulting product is nearly pure (99.5%–99.9%) and is stored as a liquefied, compressed gas at 300 psig and 4° F in insulated and refrigerated storage tanks. Figure 6-1 is a flowchart of the steps involved in manufacturing, repackaging, and distributing N_2O.

3. The manufactured product is kept refrigerated until it is directly transferred by insulated tanker trucks to hospitals with their own large storage facilities or to other gas repackagers and distributors. Approximately 3200 gas repackagers and distributors exist in the United States.[1] The dental profession stores N_2O at an estimated 83,700 locations in the United States.[1] The overall medical marketing and distribution system is very effectively and efficiently deployed in the industry.

B. Users of N_2O

1. Approximately 90% of the N_2O produced by the major manufacturing companies is used in health settings. Most of this amount (80%–85%) is used by hospitals to facilitate general anesthesia. The field of dentistry uses up to 10% of the N_2O in ambulatory clinics.[1]

2. The food industry uses approximately 5%–8% of the N_2O manufactured. N_2O acts as a propellant for dairy products such as whipped cream.[1] Nitrous oxide is dissolved within the cream until it vaporizes with ambient air when expelled from the can. Nitrous oxide produces a whipped cream that is four times the volume of the liquid. Nitrous oxide is lipophilic, thus inhibiting degradation of the fatty cream, whereas if pressurized air were used, the oxygen would cause the cream to become rancid. Nitrous oxide has also been used to displace the oxygen that causes staleness in packages of potato chips and like foods.[2]

3. The remaining users of nitrous oxide include the chemical industry, in which nitrous oxide is used in the production of sodium azide, the explosive agent that inflates an automobile air bag.

4. N_2O is used to increase engine performance in the racing industry (i.e., cars, motorcycles, boats).[1] An N_2O system is now available for personal vehicles as well.

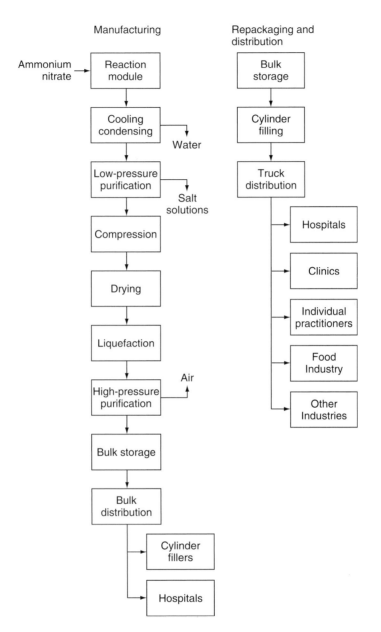

Figure 6-1 Manufacturing process and distribution of N₂0.

5. N$_2$O is also used in the silicon industry, where it oxidizes chemicals during the manu-
    facture of computer chips. This use requires a 100% pure product.[1]
6. In a hybrid rocket engine, nitrous oxide has been used as the oxidizer in combination
    with a fuel source. It has also been used in amateur and high-power rocketry.[2]

C. Manufacturers of N_2O

1. The major manufacturers of N_2O in North America are: Airgas Puritan Medical, Inc., Radnor, Pennsylvania; Air Liquide America, Houston, Texas; and AGA, Mexico City, Mexico. No US manufacturers of the small cartridges, commonly referred to as "whippets," for whipping cream dispensers are known.[2]

2. Their total output is between 30 and 35 million pounds of N_2O annually.[1]

D. Product expense

1. The entire manufacturing process is very inexpensive and provides an excellent product that is affordable for both the healthcare field and industry.

2. The cost analysis of N_2O given in Chapter 7 does not include the costs of filling, storing, maintaining, or delivering the cylinders. These costs vary geographically and depend on the volume requested by the customer, the tank size, and the distance from the manufacturing site to the customer.

II. REGULATION AND CONTROL OF NITROUS OXIDE

A. Regulatory agencies

1. The Food and Drug Administration (FDA) regulates the N_2O industry. The FDA has established Good Manufacturing Practices (GMPs) and Quality System Requirements (QSRs) with which companies who produce and package gases must comply. Compliance with these regulations results in a near 100% pure product, which exceeds U.S. Pharmacopeia specifications.

2. In addition, the U.S. Department of Transportation (DOT) oversees the packaging and transport of the gas. N_2O is considered a hazardous material because of the pressurization. Therefore, it falls under the restrictions of the DOT Hazardous Materials Regulations. Cylinders, transportation vehicles, and drivers must meet prescribed regulations. Figure 6-2 shows a truck transporting N_2O/O_2.

3. The Compressed Gas Association (CGA) and the Gases and Welding Distributors Association (GAWDA) have recommended guidelines for nitrous oxide sales and security.[3] These guidelines identify control measures that are intended to minimize

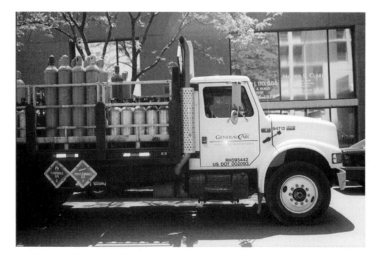

Figure 6-2 Local transportation and distribution of N_2O and O_2.

the theft of nitrous oxide and promote its legitimate use.[3] The guidelines give directives to producers, commercial carriers, repackagers and distributors, and legitimate users.[3]

B. Storing N_2O and O_2

1. Hospital settings that use bulk amounts of N_2O often store the product in large containers. These containers vary in size but range from a 3¾- to a 14-ton capacity. Obviously, economic cost savings are of greatest advantage in these situations, because the storage, handling, and refilling of cylinders are labor intensive.

2. Most often the gas is placed into smaller storage cylinders by a local distributor for delivery.

    a. The metal cylinders are imprinted with critical information, such as the origin and age of the cylinder, inspection compliance, and other important data.[4] Figure 6-3 illustrates information on the top view of typical high-pressure cylinder markings.

    b. The physical integrity of a storage cylinder determines its longevity. It is common to see cylinders 60–70 years old in distribution. Aluminum is an alternative cylinder material to alloy steel because of weight factors that affect regulation and cost of delivery. Small, fiberglass-wrapped cylinders offer a lightweight alternative for patients requiring ambulatory oxygen supplementation. These cylinders are the future trend in cylinder construction.

    c. Cylinders are color coded for easy identification. Color codes are uniform in the United States but may vary somewhat internationally (Table 6-1). However, the CGA warns that cylinder color may not be a reliable means of gas identification. Instead, the cylinder label provides a more accurate description of the contents.[5]

    d. The size of the cylinder determines the quantity of its contents. However, depending on physical properties of the gas–liquid that is compressed into the cylinder, the amounts vary. The size of the cylinder has a direct relationship with the economy of its use. Larger cylinders are more cost-effective for high-frequency use. Figure 6-4 shows examples of several different cylinder sizes. See Table 6-2 for cylinder specifications.

    e. New technology has led to the ability to more accurately track the movement of cylinders. Customers such as distributors, universities, manufacturers, and healthcare facilities can now use a handheld scanner and bar codes to monitor cylinder movement.[6]

3. Cylinder storage is important for safety reasons, as well as convenience and accessibility.

    a. One of the most important facts to remember regarding compressed gases is that under no circumstances should grease, oil, or any other lubricating substance come in contact with the gas or gas delivery equipment. Should the hydrocarbons catch fire and then contact the pressurized N_2O, a potential explosion could occur.

    b. Larger cylinders associated with a central supply system are stored in an area away from the operatory. Regulations should be followed regarding ventilating and fireproofing the storage room, as well as securing and handling the cylinders.

    c. All cylinders should be handled with care and should not be altered. Only qualified individuals should handle them.

    d. Cylinders should be secured in a place that is not readily accessible or visible to others.

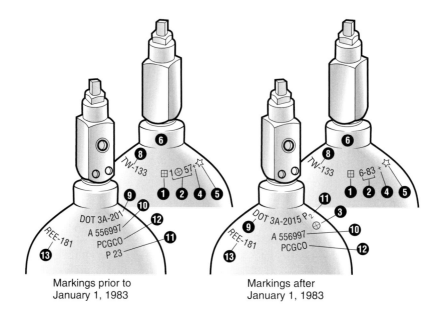

Markings prior to
January 1, 1983

Markings after
January 1, 1983

Item	Description
1	Brand identification
2	Manufacturer's test date
3	Manufacturer's registered symbol
4	Cylinder meets 10% overfill specification
5	Cylinder meets 10-year hydrostatic test exemption
6	Collar
7	Cylinder (label not shown)
8	Tare weight
9	DOT specification and service pressure
10	Manufacturer's serial number
11	Inspector's mark
12	Registered owner (PCGCO = Nellcor Puritan Bennett)
13	Rejection elastic expansion limit in cubic centimeters

Figure 6-3 Cylinder shoulder markings detailing various information.

Table 6-1. Cylinder Color Codes for Various Countries

Country	N_2O	O_2
Argentina	Blue	White with green cross
Australia	Blue	White
Canada	Blue	White
China	Gray	Blue
India	Blue	Black with white shoulders
Germany	Gray	Blue
Japan	Black	White
South Africa	Blue	Black with white shoulders
Sweden	Blue	White
United Kingdom	Blue	White
United States	Blue	Green

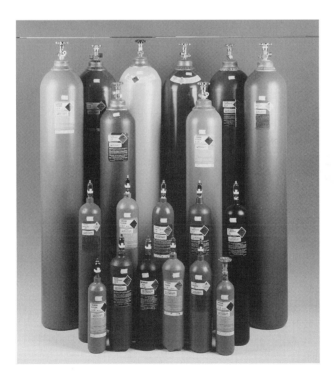

Figure 6-4 Various gas cylinder sizes. (Courtesy Nellcor Puritan Bennett.)

4. Requirements for appropriate cylinder storage, installation of equipment, etc., are found in Section 99-C of the National Fire Protection Association (NFPA) code. Additional information from the CGA and the National Welding Supply Association (NWSA) is available. See Appendix A for resources.

Table 6-2.	**Nitrous Oxide and Oxygen Cylinder Specifications***			
Common Nitrous Oxide Cylinders				
Size	Dimensions	Pressure (psig at 70° C)	Weight of N_2O	Nominal Gross Weight
D	4.25 × 17 in (10.8 × 73 cm)	745 psig	3 lb 13¼ oz (1.74 kg)	~13 lb (~2 kg)
E	4.25 × 28.75 in (10.8 ×73 cm)	745 psig	6 lb 7 oz (2.92 kg³)	~21 lb (~10 kg)
G	8.5 × 51 in (21.6 × 129.5 cm)	745 psig	56 lb (25.4 kg)	~190 lb (~86.2 kg)
H	9 × 51 in (22.9 × 129.5 cm)	745 psig	64 lb (29 kg)	~198 lb (~89.8 kg)
Common Oxygen Cylinders				
Size	Pressure (psig at 70° C)		Weight of O_2	Nominal Gross Weight
D	2015 psig		15.3 ft³ (0.42 m³)	~10 lb (~4.85 kg)
E	2015 psig		24.9 ft³ (0.69 m³)	~16.5 lb (~7.48 kg)
E (aluminum)	2015 psig		24.1 ft³ (0.67 m³)	~13 lb (~6 kg)
H	2200 psig		249 ft³ (6.9 m³)	~153 lb (~70 kg)

*Courtesy Nellcor Puritan Bennett.

C. **N_2O cylinders**
1. A full N_2O cylinder contains approximately 95% liquid and 5% vapor.
   a. Liquid N_2O in the tank is vaporized by the ambient room air temperature outside the tank as the gas is used.
   b. Because of this heat transfer process, the tank becomes cool to the touch; frost may be seen on the tank surface during prolonged and continuous use.
2. A full cylinder of N_2O will have a pressure-gauge reading of approximately 750 psi at 70° F. If the cylinder is colder as a result of storage conditions or rapid release, the full cylinder pressure will be less. At a temperature of 50° F, the cylinder pressure will be approximately 575 psi.
   a. Because the liquid is vaporized as the gas is used, this reading is not proportional to the actual amount of gas available in the cylinder.
   b. Therefore, the gauge will show a pressure decrease when the tank contains approximately 20% N_2O. The drop in the dial on the N_2O tank is not proportional to the contents of the tank as with O_2. Figure 6-5 illustrates pressure gauge readings for full and empty N_2O and O_2 cylinders.

D. **O_2 cylinders**
1. O_2 is found as a gas in a cylinder. When the O_2 cylinder is full, the amount of pressure is approximately 2000 psi.
2. The pressure gauge for O_2 will accurately indicate the amount of gas present in the cylinder at all times until the cylinder is exhausted.
   a. The dial will accurately reflect the quantity of gas available in the cylinder for use. For example, if the dial reads 1000 psi, the cylinder is considered half full.
   b. It is important to monitor the amount of O_2 left in the cylinder while it is in use. Because the N_2O/O_2 sedation machine is driven by O_2 flow, if the O_2 tank becomes empty during a procedure, there will be no flow of N_2O, and the

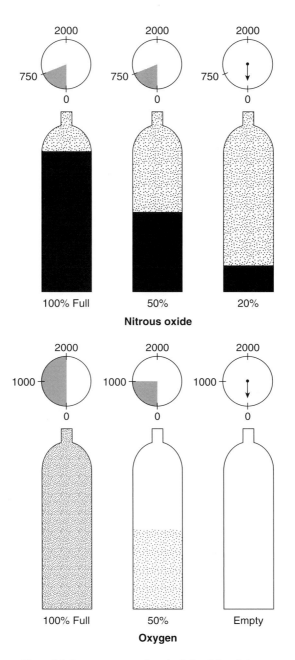

Figure 6-5 Pressure gauge readings for N_2O and O_2 cylinders.

sedation experience will be interrupted. It is important to have additional O_2 cylinders available to prevent this occurrence.

E. A 50%/50% N_2O and O_2 combination product, dispensed in a single cylinder, is manufactured under the names Kalinox and Entonox. This product is not allowed for use in the United States; however, it is used frequently in other countries.

III. MANUFACTURERS OF N_2O/O_2 SEDATION EQUIPMENT

A.   Three major companies in the United States manufacture and distribute N_2O/O_2 delivery systems. They are, in alphabetical order: Accutron, Inc., Phoenix, Arizona; Matrx by Midmark, Orchard Park, New York; and Porter Instrument Co.—A Division of Parker Hannifin Inc., Hatfield, Pennsylvania. (See Appendix A for references.)

B.   *Authors' note:* We can personally attest to the genuine concern of each of these companies to manufacture the best and safest products for the mutual benefit of both patient and clinician.

IV. DELIVERY OF N_2O/O_2

A.   **History and evolution of N_2O/O_2 delivery equipment**
1. N_2O/O_2 sedation equipment has evolved dramatically since the initial delivery through a bladder bag for Horace Wells.
2.   Sir Fredrick Hewitt in 1887 was the first to incorporate oxygen into a machine that delivered both gases.[7]
3.   Early machines were designed as intermittent (demand) flow.[7]
4.   A pivotal point in the progression of this technology was the addition of the fail-safe O_2 mechanism in the mid-1970s. This device prevented the delivery of 100% N_2O and ensured that no less than 21% O_2 (O_2 concentration in ambient air) would ever be delivered to the patient.[3] Today this tolerance is 30%.
5.   Mr. Gary Porter, president of Porter Instrument Co., Inc., played an integral role in the evolution of the early analgesia-sedation units. The Porter Instrument Co.—A Division of Parker Hannifin—is the only company to manufacture the flowmeter glass tubes found in sedation units and hospital anesthesia machines around the world.
6.   Today we enjoy the amenities of audible alarms, digital readouts, tactile-sensitive features, and high-quality performance.

B.   **Central gas supply system**
1.   A central gas supply system is used when a large quantity of gas is supplying several units. Practitioners may prefer this system because of the frequency of N_2O/O_2 use, cost savings, convenience, space saving, etc.
2.   A central-system manifold (Figure 6-6) is a device that connects several large cylinders of gas together and allows for the transfer of gas supply from one tank to another when the previous tank is depleted.
    a.   A manifold is used to connect a central gas supply to individual operatories and to ensure a constant availability of gas.
    b.   A manifold system can be manually operated or virtually be self-automated.
    c.   Manifold systems are designed to supply gas to as many as 10 units in a given facility. Beyond 10 units, the facility is considered a hospital care unit and is regulated accordingly.
    d.   The manifold system is most conveniently and effectively used when it is incorporated as part of the architectural design of the operatory (Figure 6-7).
    e.   The newest manifolds have several safety features built into the system.
        i.   Pressure-relief valves exhaust any gas higher than 75 psi.
        ii.   Alarm systems, both visual and audible, alert a designated person if the pressure of the gas falls below 45 psi or becomes greater than 60 psi. A wall alarm placed in the operatory alerts the practitioner, whereas a desk alarm alerts an individual at a central location (Figure 6-8).
3.   All gas from the manifold travels through precleaned, degreased copper tubing, and all connections are silver-soldered at 1000° F. The piping system must be pressure tested

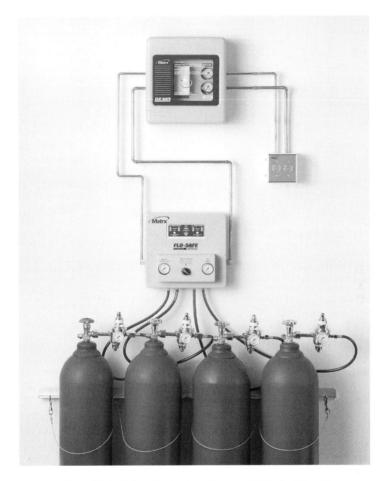

Figure 6-6 Central manifold system. *(Courtesy of Matrx by Midmark.)*

with N_2 (air) for 24 hours at no less than 150 psi before patient use. Half-inch copper tubing for delivery of O_2 and ⅜-inch tubing for N_2O have become norms. The difference in tubing size prohibits the inadvertent crossing of lines. However, at least one fatality has occurred because of installation errors and subsequent delivery of 100% N_2O instead of O_2. Piping, Industry, Progress, and Education (PIPE) is an organization dedicated to educating users of N_2O/O_2 sedation about the proper installation of the system. See Appendix A for references. *Disclaimer:* Seek professional installation of all sedation equipment to ensure all current specifications and codes are met.

4. For the gas to be dispensed safely there must be a means for reducing the amount of gas pressure from the cylinder. A pressure-reducing valve or regulator is necessary to ensure safe delivery of gas to the patient and through the equipment.

    a. The high pressures of 750 psi in the N_2O tank and 2000 psi in the O_2 tank are reduced to lower pressures of approximately 50 psi.

    b. Regulators are commonly found on or near the cylinders of central supply delivery systems.

    c. Pressure gauges accompany regulators and display gas pressures within the tank. Pressure gauges indicating the amount of pressure in the lines may also be present on a central manifold system.

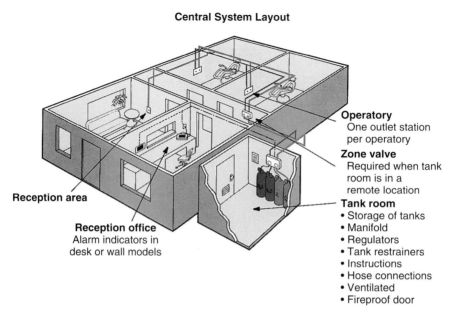

Central System Layout

Operatory
One outlet station
per operatory

Zone valve
Required when tank
room is in a
remote location

Tank room
• Storage of tanks
• Manifold
• Regulators
• Tank restrainers
• Instructions
• Hose connections
• Ventilated
• Fireproof door

Reception area

Reception office
Alarm indicators in
desk or wall models

Figure 6-7 Example of an office configuration with a central manifold system.

5. Large G and H cylinders are used in central supply systems. There is a safety feature within the threaded valves that open the cylinders. Threaded stems are designed to fit into specific cylinders only, thus preventing the cylinders from being filled with the wrong gas (Figure 6-9).

C. Portable gas delivery system

1. A portable gas delivery system is often used when N_2O/O_2 sedation is not used frequently. The unit houses smaller tanks and may be moved easily from place to place.
2. The yoke stand of the portable machine is the backbone and supporting structure on which the equipment rests. Stands vary slightly in style; all are easily transportable on wheels. Some stands hold two tanks, whereas others hold four tanks (Figure 6-10). One company markets a portable system that encloses the yoke and tanks for easy maneuverability (Figure 6-11).
3. The yoke is the metal framework adjoining the stand to which the cylinders are attached. There is an attachment configuration for the cylinder to match to be correctly attached to the unit. Metal pins, specifically arranged, protrude from the yoke onto which the cylinder is fitted (Figure 6-12). This precise mechanism is designed to prevent the incorrect cylinder attachment to the yoke and is known as the *pin index safety system* (Figure 6-13).
4. Regulators are found on portable systems similar to central delivery systems (Figure 6-14). After the gas pressure has been reduced, gas is delivered through low-pressure hosing connected to the back of the flowmeter, the boxlike portion of the unit, which contains switches, knobs, etc. (Figure 6-15). These hoses are color coded, respectively, for the gases and purposely vary in size and threaded-end connections to prevent improper gas flow to the machine.
5. At this point, the equipment is the same whether delivering gas from a central supply or a portable unit.

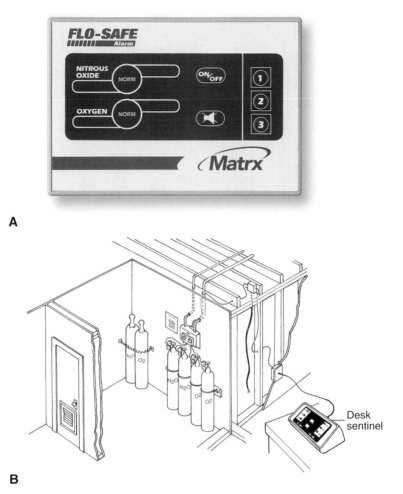

Figure 6-8 Two types of alarm systems. **A,** Wall mounted and **B,** desk mounted. *(A Courtesy of Matrx by Midmark.)*

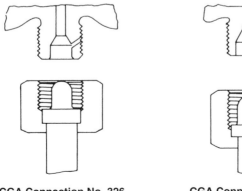

CGA Connection No. 326   CGA Connection No. 540

Figure 6-9 Large cylinder threaded valve connections.

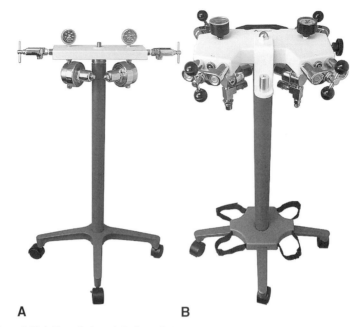

A   B

Figure 6-10 A, Two-cylinder and, **B,** four-cylinder portable yoke stands. *(Courtesy of Accutron, Inc.)*

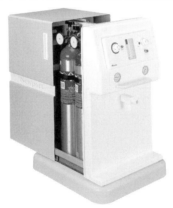

Figure 6-11 Encased portable yoke and tanks. *(Courtesy of Accutron, Inc.)*

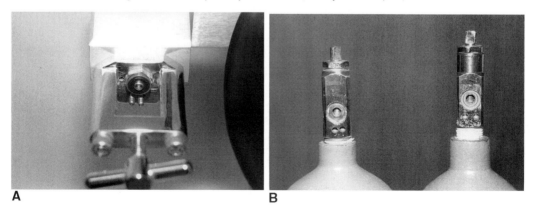

A   B

Figure 6-12 Pin index safety system. **A,** Close-up view of pins on yoke. **B,** Hole configurations; they are different depending on the cylinder's contents.

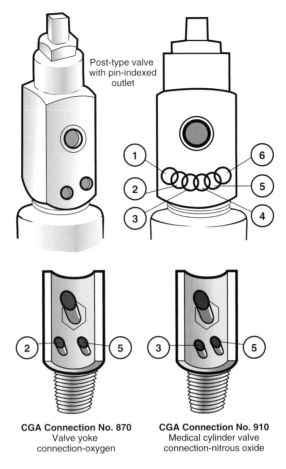

Post-type valve with pin-indexed outlet

1
2
3
6
5
4

2   5
CGA Connection No. 870
Valve yoke
connection-oxygen

3   5
CGA Connection No. 910
Medical cylinder valve
connection-nitrous oxide

Figure 6-13 Small tank pin index system.

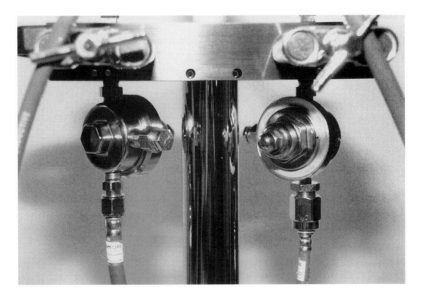

Figure 6-14 Regulators alter high pressure from cylinders to low pressure for patient delivery.

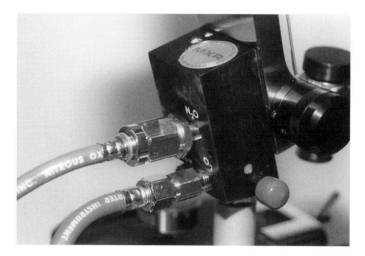

Figure 6-15 Pressure hosing from regulators into flowmeter.

D. **Flowmeter**
1. The flowmeter is the highly calibrated device that sits on top of the yoke assembly; it is mounted to the wall, or is located within the cabinetry (Figure 6-16). Gas flows from the cylinder through the flowmeter. The flowmeter indicates the amount of gas being delivered to the patient.
2. Gas flows into separate sections of the flowmeter and ultimately shows its flow in the gas tubes on the front of the unit. Small balls within the tubes rise and fall according to the amount of gas flowing into the flowmeter. The number corresponding to the middle of the ball indicates the liters of flow per minute of a gas being delivered to the patient. Digital lighted electronic displays are also available. In this case, flashing lights indicate the flow of gas (Figure 6-17, *A*). Some models show the percent of oxygen delivered, whereas others show the percent of nitrous oxide.
3. One of the most important safety features of the sedation unit is the flowmeter's fail-safe mechanism. A valve opens to allow N_2O flow only when there is flow of O_2 to the system. Any time the O_2 flow is less than 30%, N_2O stops flowing. This feature prevents the potential delivery of 100% N_2O and is standard on every sedation unit made today. *Without it, an operator is practicing below the standard of care.* See Figure 6-18 for specific features of the flowmeter.

E. **Reservoir bag**
1. The reservoir bag (Figure 6-19) serves three purposes. Its primary purpose is to provide a source of additional gas should the patient inspire more gas than is being supplied through the hoses. Typically, a reservoir bag holds approximately 3 L of gas. Other sizes are available (e.g., a smaller bag for pediatric patients).
2. In addition, the reservoir bag provides a mechanism for monitoring the patient's respiration. Watching the expansion and contraction of the bag during sedation assures the operator of the patient's quiet inhalation and exhalation.
3. The reservoir bag also functions in an emergency as a method of providing positive-pressure O_2 to the patient. The bag is gently squeezed to empty its contents into the pulmonary tree; the action is similar to a manual-resuscitator bag. Assisting ventilation in this manner overcomes resistance when accompanied by a full-face mask with a tight seal rather than a nasal hood.

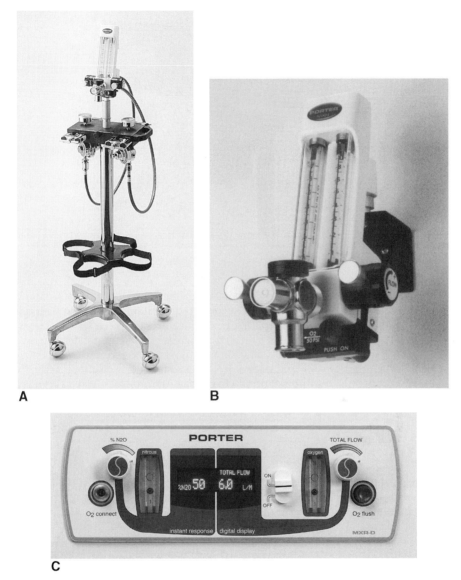

Figure 6-16 A, Flowmeter on top of yoke assembly. **B,** Flowmeter mounted to wall. **C,** Flowmeter located within cabinetry. *(Courtesy of Porter Instrument Co.—A Division of Parker Hannifin.)*

F.   Conduction tubing

1.   Gas is delivered through tubing or hose stemming from the unit and attaching to the breathing apparatus, as shown in Figure 6-20.
2.   Care should be taken to prevent kinking of the hose, thereby preventing gas flow. If this should happen, the patient will most likely alert the operator of breathing difficulty. The reservoir bag will also overfill and balloon because of the constriction of the hose.

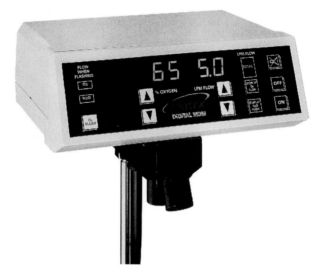

Figure 6-17 Digital LED flowmeter. *(Courtesy of Matrx by Midmark.)*

3. The concept of anatomic dead space is related to the length of the conduction tubing. This space will contain gas that neither gets into the pulmonary tree to be used nor is expelled from the system to be replaced by fresh gas, hence "dead space." The distance from the gas source to the patient's lungs can increase the anatomic dead space and be lengthened by the conduction tubing. It is important not to add hose to facilitate delivery to another area or the other side of the room because of this factor.

4. Units may consist of a combination of corrugated and noncorrugated tubing. Tubing diameters vary, with most tubing narrowing near the attachment of the breathing apparatus.

5. Currently manufactured conduction tubing is latex free, whereas previously manufactured products may not be. Check with the product representative for information about existing products.

G. Breathing apparatus (nasal hood or face mask)

1. Gas may be delivered to the patient through a nasal hood or a full-face mask. Nitrous oxide and oxygen are typically delivered via a nasal hood. All currently manufactured nasal hoods are latex free, whereas previously manufactured products may not be. Check with the product representative for information about existing products.

2. The nasal hood is most commonly used with today's sedation equipment. One of the reasons for this is that dentistry represents a large sample of the product consumers.

   a. The nasal hood is designed to fit snugly over the patient's nose so that gas does not leak out the sides. Several sizes are available (Figure 6-21).

   b. Hoods are offered in a variety of scents, such as vanilla, peach, strawberry, mint, and bubble gum (Figure 6-22). Unscented nasal hoods are also available.

   c. The most current models of nasal hoods are designed for single patient use. Many regard these as disposable because they are not sterilizable. Other reusable versions of the hoods are also available but must be sterilized between patients (Figure 6-23).

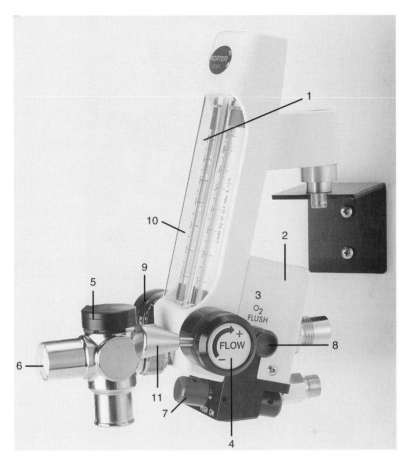

Figure 6-18 Flowmeter features. *1,* Flowmeter tubes; *2,* fail-safe; *3,* gas control block; *4,* gas flow adjustment knobs; *5,* emergency air valve; *6,* check valve (nonrebreathing valve); *7,* positive ON-OFF switch; *8,* oxygen flush button; *9,* needle valves; *10,* flowmeter; *11,* total flow adjustment knob. *(Courtesy of Porter Instrument Co.—A Division of Parker Hannifin.)*

    d. Practitioners may choose to dispose of the nasal hood and recover the cost in the sedation fee or sell the nasal hood to patients and suggest they bring it to the next appointment.

    e. All nasal hoods should have scavenging capabilities. Scavenging nasal hoods are designed to provide fresh gas to the hood for the patient through two hoses, while one or two additional hoses evacuate gas being exhaled by the patient (see Figure 6-24). These hoses are connected to a vacuum system that exhausts the gases out of the building.

    f. *It is considered practicing below the standard of care for any healthcare provider not to use a scavenging nasal hood.*

3. A full-face mask may be used in place of the nasal hood when accessibility to the mouth is not an issue. Because the mask is intended to cover both the mouth and nose, it is much larger than the nasal hood. Patients may remark that it is claustrophobic by design and may be more anxious about its placement. It is generally used for anesthetic procedures (i.e., general anesthesia) or emergency oxygen delivery (see Figure 6-25).

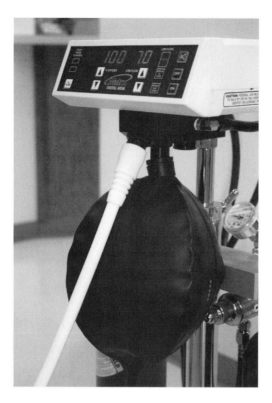

Figure 6-19 Reservoir bag.

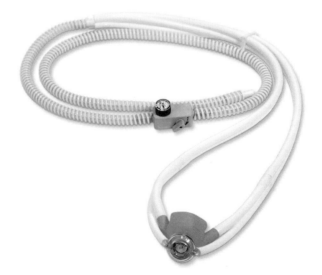

Figure 6-20 Conduction tubing connected to scavenging nasal hood. *(Courtesy of Accutron, Inc.)*

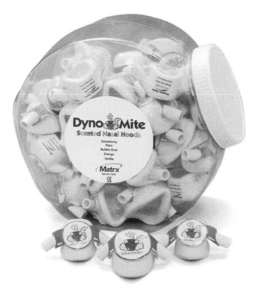

Figure 6-21 Scavenging nasal hoods in a variety of sizes. *(Courtesy of Matrx by Midmark.)*

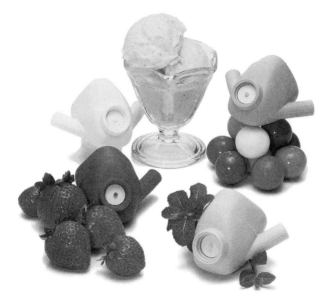

Figure 6-22 Scavenging nasal hoods in a variety of scents. *(Courtesy of Accutron, Inc.)*

V. VARIATIONS OF EQUIPMENT

A. Design

1. Currently, a variety of available designs of sedation equipment from which to choose are available. Manufacturers determine their own style, color, size, etc., of equipment. However, the design features are similar. Each has common performance features and similar safety features; any variations are in location of the features on the equipment and whether they are manual or automatic.

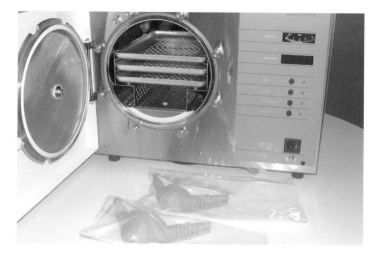

Figure 6-23 Some scavenging nasal hoods are sterilizable and can be reused. *(Courtesy of Porter Instrument Co.—A Division of Parker Hannifin.)*

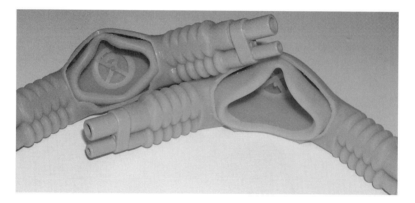

Figure 6-24 Two hoses bring fresh gas while two hoses evacuate exhaled gas.

2. A sedation unit may have separate controls (Figure 6-26), one regulating the flow of N_2O and another controlling O_2 flow. In this case, both knobs will be used as the gases are delivered.

3. Another type of unit (Figure 6-27) mixes the gases together and controls the total flow being delivered to a patient. Once tidal volume is established, this unit is designed to maintain a constant total flow to the patient; the mixture of gas (percentage of nitrous oxide) is then increased or decreased by use of one knob or button.

4. All U.S. companies have designed digital sedation units; their features may be slightly different from each other; however, each includes an LED panel (Figure 6-28). The mixing unit is controlled with arrow keys for increasing or decreasing gas, and it can maintain a constant liter flow. This machine has many advantages, such as automaticity and precision of gas flow. Some units have audible alarms. These units may be flush-mounted, attached to a swing arm, or on a portable yoke system.

5. The Ultra flowmeter, designed by Accutron, Inc., has the capability of blocking the flow of N_2O with a lock. This feature maintains the value of the machine as an

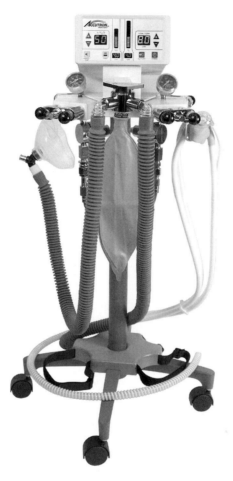

Figure 6-25 Unit with full-face mask. *(Courtesy of Accutron, Inc.)*

O_2-delivering mechanism in emergency situations while simultaneously securing the N_2O. This company has also introduced a remote control that is capable of remotely increasing or decreasing nitrous oxide or flow to the unit (see Figure 6-29). In addition, a small machine is available that will print out the flow of gases and the percent of nitrous oxide administered on a small piece of paper that can be placed in the patient's chart as partial documentation of the procedure (see Figure 6-30).

6. An international manufacturer in Japan produces a machine that calculates the amount of N_2O and O_2 used for a procedure. The cost of N_2O is quite high in Japan. Consumers are charged for the exact amount (per gram) of N_2O used. The machine displays the amount and subsequent charge to the patient on a receiptlike slip of paper for direct reimbursement to the healthcare facility (see Chapter 7).

B. Customization

1. Depending on specific consumer needs, manufacturers can customize equipment accordingly.
2. Restrictions may apply regarding the maximum allowable N_2O concentrations able to be administered by some groups, countries, or organizations. Certain military groups

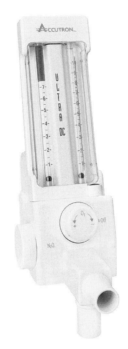

Figure 6-26 Sedation unit with separate gas flow controls. *(Courtesy of Accutron, Inc.)*

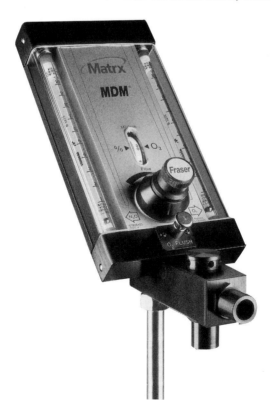

Figure 6-27 Sedation unit capable of mixing gases and maintaining constant tidal volume. *(Courtesy of Matrx by Midmark.)*

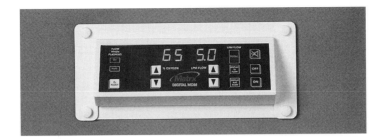

Figure 6-28 Wall-mounted digital LED panel. *(Courtesy of Matrx by Midmark.)*

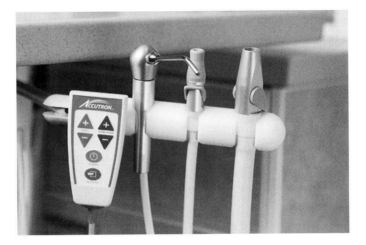

Figure 6-29 Remote control to sedation unit. *(Courtesy of Accutron, Inc.)*

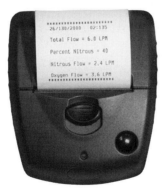

Figure 6-30 Printout of flow and percentage of nitrous oxide administered. *(Courtesy of Accutron, Inc.)*

regulate concentrations and thus purchase units that have been customized to limit the amount of N$_2$O able to be delivered.

3. Equipment available for international use varies widely. Depending on the country that uses the sedation equipment, markings may be customized to accommodate various languages; colored hoses, tubing, etc., may vary depending on the color codes specific to a country.

C. Cost

1. The cost of the necessary sedation equipment should not be prohibitive to providing this service. Expenses will be recovered quickly with patient use and reimbursement of fees. The production and administrative costs associated with N_2O/O_2 sedation remain relatively low. It is still extremely economical and profitable to deliver N_2O/O_2 sedation in the ambulatory setting. See Chapter 7 for more information on the economic benefits.

2. As mentioned previously, it is necessary to choose the delivery mode according to the frequency of use. A central system is much more cost-effective; it should be included in building plans if frequent use is expected. The portable system offers the flexibility of moving from place to place without the initial expense.

3. Although initial costs for the central system are much greater than for the portable system, the use of N_2O provides economic benefit. The greater initial cost of the central system can be recovered in a short time.

D. Maintenance

1. Manufacturers recommend servicing sedation units periodically. Each company may have specific time frames for maintenance of its units. It is prudent to follow these recommendations to ensure safe delivery to the patient.

2. Servicing a unit includes procedures such as recalibration, pressure testing, internal component checking and replacement, and other factory testing procedures.

3. If at any time the integrity of the equipment is questionable or the unit is not functioning properly, it is important to discontinue its use and alert those who service the equipment. Unqualified personnel must not be allowed to tamper with or attempt to repair any sedation equipment. Servicing and inspecting must be left to those who are properly trained.

VI. EQUIPMENT SAFETY FEATURES

A. Several safety features are inherent components of N_2O/O_2 delivery equipment for ambulatory settings. These features provide both patient and professional assurance of the safe delivery of N_2O/O_2 sedation.

1. The most important safety feature of the unit is the O_2 fail-safe mechanism. It ensures that N_2O will not be delivered unless there is O_2 flowing to the machine. Because of this device, the possibility of administering 100% N_2O to a patient has been eliminated. The mechanism's function is based on pressure. O_2 flows into the unit at a pressure that opens a valve to allow the flow of N_2O. If the O_2 pressure drops because of depletion of the supply, the valve closes, thereby preventing the flow of N_2O. This safety feature is standard on every sedation unit manufactured today. Units made before 1976, when this feature was added, should not be used. The use of outdated equipment places operators in legal jeopardy, because they are practicing below the established standard of care.

2. Currently, the units manufactured in the United States are designed to deliver a minimum of 30% O_2 at all times. It is critical to maintain an O_2 level of at least that in ambient air (21%). The minimum of 30% established by the manufacturers allows for a margin of error in calibration. Similarly, the equipment is designed to deliver no more than 70% N_2O at any time. For analgesia and sedation purposes, it is not necessary to administer N_2O concentrations higher than 70%.

3. An index safety system is designed to prevent the inadvertent attachment of the N_2O cylinder to an O_2 portal.

    a. A pin system is used for portable machines in which small cylinders attach to the yoke. Each cylinder of compressed gas has two small holes drilled into the valve stem that correspond to a specific configuration identifying the contents of the cylinder. Two small pins on each portal of the yoke configured exactly with the holes on the cylinder form the attachment mechanism between the cylinder and unit (see Figure 6-12).

   b. On equipment that uses larger tanks, the index system includes thread size and configuration of the valve connection on the tank to the regulator. Again, each gas has a specific configuration to avoid incorrect attachments (see Figure 6-9).

4. With the diameter index safety system, the hoses through which the gas travels from the cylinder to the unit are unable to be attached to the wrong stem. The attachment couplings are different in diameter, as are the hoses and stems (Figure 6-31).

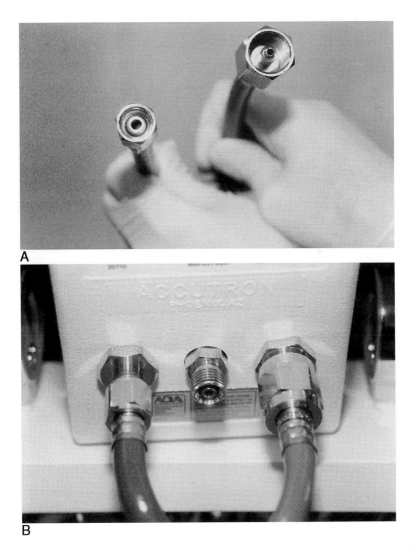

Figure 6-31 A, Note the difference in diameter of the attachment couplings in the diameter safety system. **B,** Improper attachment is avoided with the diameter index safety system.

5. Near the unit's reservoir bag is an emergency air inlet. This provides an additional source of air for the patient in the circumstance that the reservoir bag is inadequate or the gas flow decreases for some reason (see Figure 6-18).
6. A nonrebreathing valve located near the reservoir bag prohibits exhaled gas from the tubing from entering the reservoir bag (see Figure 6-18).
7. The reservoir bag may serve to assist with patient respirations should an emergency situation arise.
8. There is an auxiliary positive-pressure oxygen hookup on the unit capable of accommodating a quick-connect bag and mask (Figure 6-32). The sedation unit is indispensable for emergency medical situations.

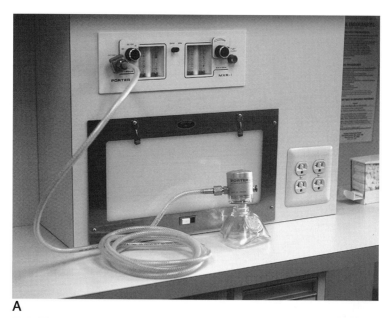

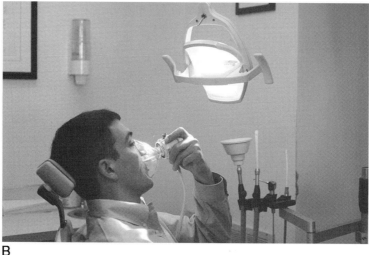

Figure 6-32 A and **B,** Positive-pressure oxygen connection with quick-connect mask for emergency situations. *(Courtesy of Porter Instrument Co.—A Division of Parker Hannifin.)*

9. Several alarm options exist, depending on the type of system or unit being used. Alarms can be audible and/or visual to indicate a depleting oxygen supply. Audible alarms are mandatory in Europe and are recommended in the United States.

REFERENCES

1. Compressed Gas Association: Nitrous oxide fact sheet, *http://cganet.com/N2O/factsht.asp*, 2006.
2. Nitrous oxide: *http://answers.com*, 2006.
3. Compressed Gas Association: Nitrous oxide sales and security recommended guidelines, *http://cganet.com/N2O/guidelin.asp*, 2006.
4. Compressed Gas Association: *CGA G-8.2–2000 Commodity Specification for Nitrous Oxide*, ed 4, Arlington, VA, 2000, The Association.
5. Compressed Gas Association: *CGA Code-9, Standard Color Marking of Compressed Gas Containers Intended for Medical Use*, Arlington, VA, 1993, The Association.
6. Linweld, Inc.: The Medical Gas Monitor: Cylinder tracking aids asset management, Vol. 5, Fall 2005, Linweld Inc.
7. Malamed SF: *Sedation: A Guide to Patient Management*, ed 4, St. Louis, 2003, Mosby.

Chapter 7

Economic Benefits Associated with N₂O/O₂ Administration

When the subject of economics enters the realm of patient care, many practitioners begin to feel uneasy. Although financial expectations may not be the centerpiece of a decision to pursue a health career, they often are a significant factor. Being financially successful is not unethical by itself, although there are those in the medical profession who have abused the system for financial gain. However, nothing is wrong with caring about people and enjoying the benefits of success. Health professionals should feel good about the services they provide and be profitable enough to continue to practice them.

I. ECONOMIC REFLECTION

A. The "Golden Age of Medicine and Dentistry," a period of post–World War II prosperity that lasted into the early 1960s, was a time of high demand for services and a shortage of clinicians. This situation assured professionals that their practices would be profitable. Because patients were waiting at the door, schedules became tight and profits became palpable. Unfortunately, time and compassion for the patient were not as important for many as they should have been.

B. As the supply of practitioners began to increase in the early 1970s, the demand for healthcare professionals decreased, as did the patient/practitioner ratio.

C. Renewed interest in the relationship between clinician and patient has demanded greater sensitivity to patient problems, payment plans, and scheduling demands, and an overall awareness of patient needs.

II. REALISTIC ECONOMICS

A. Today's patients have a greater choice in the overall environment of treatment. If they are not treated considerately in one office, they can more easily than ever find an office that makes a greater effort toward meeting their individual needs. This is the basic economic principle of supply and demand in action. Caring, compassionate, competent practitioners are doing very well and have not had economic setbacks because of "too much competition." Indeed, choice has led to patient sophistication in consumerism.

B. Regardless of the socioeconomic strata or educational profiles of patients, they as human beings can easily, quickly, and accurately recognize the sincerity of a clinician. On the basis of experiences, patients use their intuition to determine whether they will continue with a certain doctor and whether they will refer others to that doctor. Patients do not necessarily have the ability to evaluate a clinician's technical or decision-making skills; therefore, their evaluations are based on the clinicians' personal interactions with them.

C. With the advent of managed care, health maintenance organizations (HMOs), preferred provider organization (PPO) programs, and changing insurance issues, practitioners' knowledge and understanding of economics becomes critical to survival. Clearly, ambulatory services have and will continue to increase because of the regulations placed on time, payments, extent of treatment, etc. Many practitioners believe that these issues have become so intrusive that patient care has suffered.

D.   The tremendous overall transformation in medical/dental practice is challenging practitioners to find new avenues for providing patient care with renewed compassion. They may have to advocate services in a different manner. Practitioners may have to rethink their commitment to the profession and to the patient. They may have to become innovative in treatment planning.

E.   Patients are always grateful for honest and sincere efforts. In time, they will demand the return of lost services and individual decision making. They will stand behind those professionals they trust. Practices are truly patient driven.

III. DOLLARS AND "SENSE"

A.   Do you consider your patients' comfort levels valuable? Are you less stressed because you have relaxed, cooperative patients? If so, how much money is that worth? Although these and other rhetorical questions may be intangible, a more concrete question is "How much money can you truly save or earn with N_2O/O_2 sedation in your practice?" Box 7-1 shows the income potential of the use of N_2O/O_2 sedation.

B.   The actual cost savings or moneymaking potential of the use of N_2O/O_2 sedation varies with certain factors. Patient numbers will increase, and time efficiency will be enhanced. These factors alone will increase bottom-line figures proportionally.

   1.   An initial decision must be made as to what type of N_2O/O_2 system will be the most beneficial and cost-effective. Table 7-1 compares the central gas supply system with the portable gas supply system.

      a.   Obviously, if N_2O/O_2 sedation will be common practice in a particular setting, a central supply system should be considered.

         i.   This system allows for multiple flowmeters to be placed in several rooms. Piping and connecting are done within the structure; therefore, moving machines and hoses from room to room is not necessary.

         ii. This type of system allows for larger quantities of gas to be stored in a remote location. Larger cylinders, capable of storing more gas, are much less expensive per unit of gas than smaller ones.

      b.   Individual, portable units are also available. Practitioners may choose this option as a personal preference, especially when they only occasionally use

---

Box 7-1   INCOME POTENTIAL WITH N_2O/O_2 SEDATION

Weekly:	**Monthly:**
Twice per week = $100	Twice per week = $400
Once per day = $250	Once per day = $1000
Twice per day = $500	Twice per day = $2000
	Yearly:
	Once per day = $12,000

NOTE: Fees for N_2O/O_2 sedation range from $50–$120 per visit. Figures based on $50 and E cylinders.

Table 7-1. Tank Size Cost Comparison

Cylinder Type	Gas	Tank Capacity (Liters)	Cost per Tank	Cost per Liter	1/2 Hour Procedure					Total Gas Usage		Cost	Patients per Week	Weeks per Year	Total Procedures	Cost
					Gas Delivery	Total Minutes	Gas	LPM	Total Gas LPM	Gas	LPM	Total Cost				
E	O₂	625	$16.00	$0.026	Initial	5	O₂	6	30	O₂	120	$3.07				
E	N₂O	1590	$31.00	$0.019	Procedure	20	N₂O	3	60	N₂O	60	$1.17				
					Procedure	20	O₂	3	60							
					Postoxygen	5	O₂	6	30							

E Cylinder Tank

		Total Cost	Patients per Week	Weeks per Year	Total Procedures	Cost
1/2 Hr Procedure		$4.24	20	45	900	$3817.63
	O₂	120	$0.40			
	N₂O	60	$0.38			

Cylinder Type	Gas	Tank Capacity (Liters)	Cost per Tank	Cost per Liter	Gas Delivery	Total Minutes	Gas	LPM	Total Gas LPM
H & G	O₂	6907	$23.00	$0.003	Initial	5	O₂	6	30
H & G	N₂O	13,884	$87.00	$0.006	Procedure	20	N₂O	3	60
					Procedure	20	O₂	3	60
					Postoxygen	5	O₂	6	30

H & G Cylinder Tank

	Total Cost	Patients per Week	Weeks per Year	Total Procedures	Cost
1/2 Hr Procedure	$0.78	20	45	900	$698.01
Savings	$3.47		Savings		$3,119.62

Nitrous Revenue			
$25 Fee	$ 22,500	Profit	$ 21,802
$40 Fee	$ 36,000	Profit	$ 35,302

(Courtesy of Mr. Mike Lynam, Porter Instrument, Co.—A Division of Parker Hannifin.)

N₂O/O₂ and when confines of the physical structure do not allow for a central system.

    i. The entire portable system is on a rolling stand and may be moved from room to room.

    ii. Gas cylinders for this type of system are smaller, store less gas, and are more expensive per unit of gas than gas cylinders for central systems.

  c. In either situation, the initial cost of the N₂O/O₂ equipment should not be a prohibiting factor for its use. This investment will be quickly recovered.

2. The cost of N₂O and O₂ gases varies considerably in terms of size and quantity of cylinders ordered and distance from a distribution center. Depending on location, costs increase proportionally to the levels of individuals involved with distributorship. Gas costs will most likely be higher the further the distance from a distributor (Figure 7-1).

3. Patient charges for N₂O/O₂ sedation vary dramatically. They can range from $50 per visit to $120 per visit.

  a. Some professionals do not charge the patient for N₂O/O₂ sedation but rather include it in the overall fee for service to the patient.

  b. Insurance companies vary as to their payment policies for this service. It is wise to investigate what is considered to be the usual and customary fee according to your most common insurance carriers and local practitioners. The American

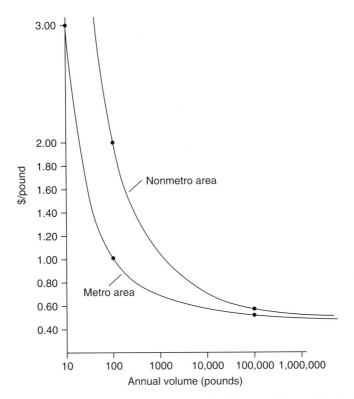

Figure 7-1 Medical N₂O pricing, metropolitan areas versus nonmetropolitan areas. *(Courtesy Nelcor Puritan Bennett.)*

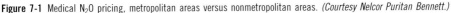

Dental Association's (ADA) Code on Dental Procedures and Nomenclature is contained in the CDT user guide. The maintenance of these codes is the responsibility of the Council on Dental Benefit Programs with consultation from Blue Cross and Blue Shield Association, the Health Insurance Association of America, the Health Care Financing Association, National Electronic Information Corporation, and the ADA recognized dental specialty organizations. Similar codes are available from the American Medical Association as current procedural terminology (CPT). The current ADA code number for analgesia, anxiolysis, or inhalation of nitrous oxide is D9230.

    c. In Japan, an N_2O/O_2 machine has the ability to determine the amount of gas delivered to the patient in terms of "flow time." The charge to the patient is calculated according to the cost of the gas multiplied by the amount of gas used. The machine is capable of printing out a charge slip for the patient at each visit (Figure 7-2).

C. Although dollar figures vary between individual situations, N_2O/O_2 sedation is profitable. Figures relating to profit in goodwill from acknowledging and diminishing patients' anxiety should not be discounted. Profit is also made by patient referrals. In economic jargon, this is a win-win situation. It just makes sense.

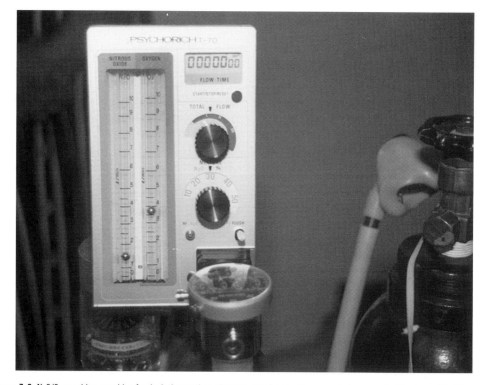

Figure 7-2 N_2O/O_2 machine capable of calculating patient charges according to the amount of gas used. *(Courtesy of Dr. Yuzuru Kaneko, Dept. of Dental Anesthesiology, Tokyo Dental College, Tokyo, Japan.)*

Part II

ANATOMY, PHYSIOLOGY, AND ADMINISTRATION

Anatomy and Physiology of Respiration and Airway Management

A ny method of inhalation sedation involves those anatomic structures associated with the inhalation and exhalation of air and the exchange of gases. To integrate the pharmacologic properties of N_2O into a clinical setting, the basic principles of the anatomy and physiology of respiration should be reviewed.

I. THE RESPIRATORY SYSTEM DESIGN AND FUNCTION

A. Design. The respiratory system is primarily designed to perform the function of exchanging gases—functionally carbon dioxide (CO_2) and O_2—across pulmonary capillary membranes. The design of the system allows this function to be performed continuously and with minimal effort by the body.[1]

B. Function. Respiration is primarily driven at two anatomical sites—automatically by the brainstem (medulla oblongata) and voluntarily by the cerebral cortex.[2]

II. THE ANATOMY OF THE UPPER AIRWAY

A. Nose
1. N_2O enters the respiratory tree at the nose.
2. The respiratory functions of the nose are to warm incoming air to body temperature, to humidify the air, and to filter macroparticles by means of nose hair and microparticles by means of cilia.
3. Because the nose is also a primary entrance for gases used during inhalation sedation, it is critical to the effectiveness of the procedure that a patient is able to breathe well. Anatomic conditions affecting air passage through the nose (e.g., a deviated septum, enlarged tonsils, and adenoids) may interfere with N_2O/O_2 delivery.

B. Pharynx
1. The pharynx is a cylindrical, muscular tube approximately 12–14 cm long.
2. It is divided into three sections (Figure 8-1): the nasopharynx, oropharynx, and laryngopharynx.
    a. The nasopharynx is located behind the nasal cavity. The adenoids, tonsils, and openings to the eustachian tubes are found here. The soft palate separates the nasopharynx from the oropharynx.
    b. The oropharynx opens into the mouth and serves as the link between the nasopharynx and the laryngopharynx. It serves as an entrance to the larynx and esophagus. Its boundaries are the soft palate and the epiglottis at the level of the hyoid bone. The epiglottis is connected by the medial glossoepiglottic fold and bilateral glossoepiglottic fold. These folds create a depression called the *valleculae*. Lateral to this central area on either side is a piriform recess. These recesses are the

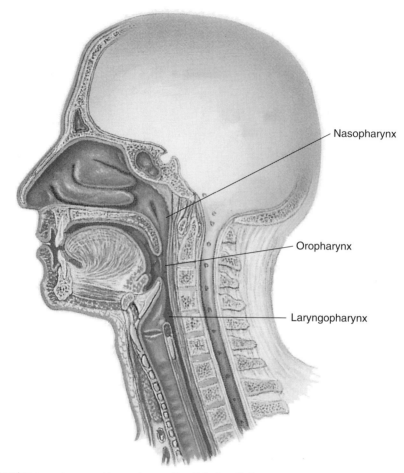

Figure 8-1 Nasopharynx, oropharynx, and laryngopharynx. *(From Thibodeau GA, Patton KT: Anatomy and Physiology, ed 6, St. Louis, 2007, Mosby.)*

      common location for collecting foreign objects in the upper airway, thereby protecting the lower airway.

   c. The laryngopharynx begins at the epiglottis. The epiglottis is the cartilaginous, leaf-shaped structure that projects upward behind the tongue. This flaplike structure (Figure 8-2) directs material backward to the esophagus and prevents objects from entering the trachea during swallowing. The laryngopharynx extends from the epiglottis to the cricoid cartilage. The larynx lies inside the laryngopharynx. The framework of the laryngopharynx is made up of the thyroid cartilage, which is shaped like a shield, and the cricoid cartilage, which is ring-shaped. Several muscle groups and ligaments cover these large structures. Both cartilages offer significant protection to the underlying larynx.

III. THE ANATOMY OF THE LOWER AIRWAY

A.　Larynx

   1. The air passageway continues with the larynx. Pearl-colored vocal cords are housed here, which, when vibrated with air, produce vocal sound. The glottal opening at the

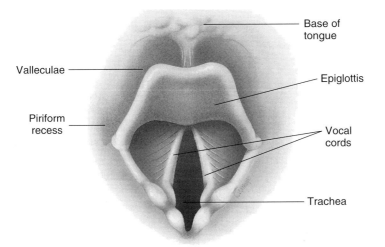

Base of tongue

Valleculae

Epiglottis

Piriform recess

Vocal cords

Trachea

Figure 8-2 Larynx and epiglottis. *(From Thibodeau GA, Patton KT:* Anatomy and Physiology, *ed 6, St. Louis, 2007, Mosby.)*

vocal cords is the narrowest part of the adult airway; the cricoid ring is the narrowest part of the pediatric (younger than 7–10 years of age) airway.

2. Strong muscles (false vocal cords) that adduct to prevent entry of foreign objects protect the sensitive mucosa of the larynx. If the larynx is irritated, the defensive cough reflex is initiated. Coughing occurs when high pressure is produced in the lower respiratory tract by the closing epiglottis and vocal cords and the contracting expiratory and abdominal muscles. A sudden opening of the false vocal cords allows the air to explode out of the respiratory tract, carrying the foreign matter with it.[2] It is important to note that when N_2O is used appropriately, this vital defensive reflex remains intact.

B. Trachea

1. The trachea, a muscular tube contiguous with the larynx, begins at the sixth cervical vertebra and is surrounded by horseshoe-shaped cartilaginous rings. It is approximately 11 cm long with a lumen size of approximately 20 mm. Figure 8-3 shows the trachea and bronchi.

2. The trachea bifurcates asymmetrically into the right and left bronchi. A highly sensitive, neurologically rich area, the carina (Figure 8-4), marks this bifurcation. The carina is considered a backup defense mechanism for the cough reflex. If an object passes through the first defensive site (larynx), the carina will initiate an even stronger cough reflex secondarily. Submucosal swelling and partial obstruction in this area can result from a strong stimulus and lead to severe airway resistance.

C. Bronchi

1. The right bronchus is approximately 2.5 cm long and deviates slightly from the trachea at approximately 25 degrees. Because of the minimal divergence from the trachea, aspirated foreign objects are more commonly directed to the right lung. Comparatively, the left bronchus is twice as long and smaller in diameter than its right counterpart. It deviates closer to 45 degrees from the trachea (see Figure 8-4).

2. The mainstem bronchi diverge into smaller branches responsible for the upper, middle, and lower lobes of the lung. The right bronchus divides into three branches, which link to three upper lobes, two middle lobes, and five lower lobes. The left bronchus

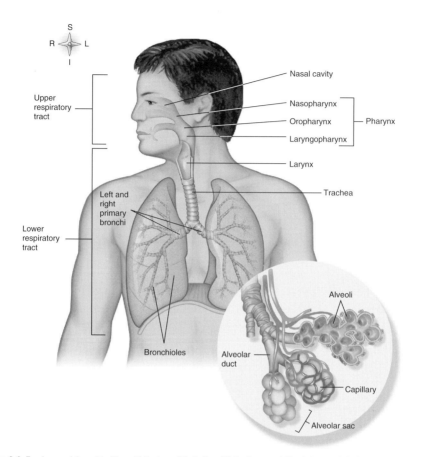

Figure 8-3 Trachea and bronchi. *(From Thibodeau GA, Patton KT:* Anatomy and Physiology, *ed 6, St. Louis, 2007, Mosby.)*

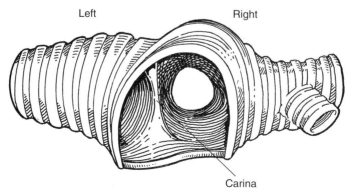

Figure 8-4 Carina located at the bifurcation of the bronchi.

bifurcates into two branches that give rise to five upper lobes and four lower lobes. Each lobe contains conducting and respiratory bronchioli with dependent alveolar ducts, sacs, and alveoli.

D. Bronchioles
   1. Bronchioles are a continued division of the bronchi but are identified by the lack of cartilage.
   2. The first 16 of the 23 generations of bronchiole divisions are considered conducting airways in normal anatomy.[2] These airways are incapable of exchanging gases. At generation 17 the respiratory bronchioli begin the respiratory zone. These are smaller than the parent bronchioli but contain significantly more surface area.[2]

IV. THE ANATOMY OF THE RESPIRATORY ZONE

A. Bronchioli, alveolar ducts, alveolar sacs, and alveoli
   1. Alveolar ducts mark the transition between bronchioli, alveolar sacs, and alveoli, as shown in Figure 8-3.
   2. Alveolar sacs "pouch" to form the thin-walled alveoli.
   3. It is in the 300 million alveoli of an adult that the exchange between air and blood takes place.[2]

V. THE PHYSIOLOGY OF THE RESPIRATORY MECHANISM

A. The medullary center in the brainstem controls the automatic respiratory process of breathing. Active inspiration is accomplished principally by the diaphragm and external intercostal muscles and assisted by the scalenes and sternocleidomastoids. As the diaphragm moves downward, the chest wall expands, creating negative pressure in the pleural space, thereby allowing a vacuum effect to pull air into the system. This motion, producing a drop in air pressure in the lungs, provides the principal mechanics for inspiration.

B. Air continues to flow until pressures from inside the lung are equivalent to atmospheric pressure. Expiration occurs passively as the chest wall and lungs recoil. This recoil causes another pressure change in which the compressed air is quietly pushed out of the lungs. Expiration becomes active only when changes in respiratory demands, such as exercise, abnormalities, or disease, occur. This automatic, regular ebb-and-flow movement of air is called tidal flow because of its similarities to that of the ocean tide.[2]

C. Because of the pressure gradient that exists between the lung walls and the thoracic cavity, the lungs are distended and fill the cavity while atmospheric pressure pushes the chest wall inward. The fluid between the structures prevents the two from separating. If air enters the pleural cavity, as in a trauma, a pneumothorax results. The fluid holding the lungs against the wall cannot hold the two together.

D. The amount of gas inspired into the lungs (tidal volume) depends largely on the physical characteristics of the individual (Figure 8-5). Generally, larger chest cavities hold more volume than smaller chest cavities. Males' lung volumes are approximately 25% greater than those of females in general.[3]
   1. In a normal-sized adult of average physical ability and without lung disease, the tidal volume approaches 500 ml. Minute ventilation (volume) is the amount of gas brought into the lungs each minute. It is calculated by multiplying the tidal volume by the rate of respiration (e.g., 500 ml $\times$ 12–15 respirations per minute = approximately 6–7 L/min).[1-3]
   2. Minute ventilation is significant in terms of N_2O administration, because it deals with how much gas mixture (N_2O/O_2) should be given to a patient. Inadequate amounts are likely to produce a suffocating feeling and make the act of breathing laborious.

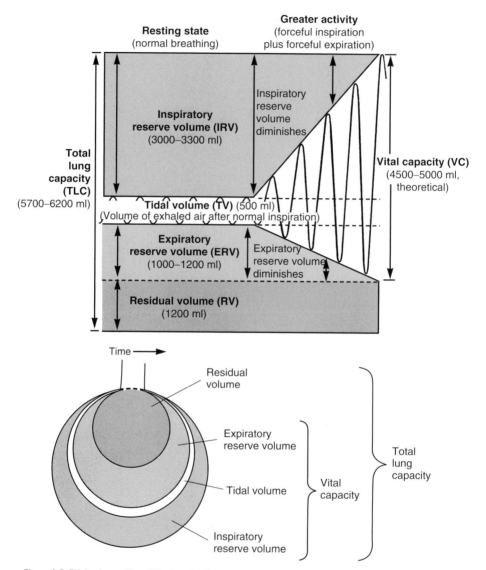

Figure 8-5 Tidal volume. *(From Thibodeau GA, Patton KT:* Anatomy and Physiology, *ed 6, St. Louis, 2007, Mosby.)*

Conversely, too much gas forced into the nasal hood of the delivery system will cause some to be wasted. The gas will escape, because it is not being consumed by the patient. This excess airflow not only blows into the patient's eyes, causing dryness, but also exposes personnel to unnecessary amounts of trace gas.

3. Alveolar ventilation is the amount of air per minute entering the alveolar units capable of gas–blood exchange. This volume is less than the minute volume, because not all of the inspired air reaches the alveoli during inspiration. A portion of the inhaled air occupies the conducting airways and does not enter the lungs and, therefore, is not taken up into the exhaust system. Hence, this air is not able to participate in the gas–blood exchange. This is known as anatomic dead space. Therefore, alveolar

ventilation is calculated by subtracting the dead space volume (approximately 150 ml) from the tidal volume and then multiplying by the respiration rate.[3]

E. The critical gas exchange from alveolus to capillary and vice versa occurs through simple diffusion across partial-pressure gradients.
   1. Atmospheric air is composed of 79.02% N_2, 20.94% O_2, and 0.04% CO_2. Other gases are negligible (Box 8-1). Combined, these gases produce a pressure of 760 mm Hg at sea level. Each component in the atmosphere does not exert the same amount of pressure. The individual gas pressure is known as partial pressure.
   2. A gas dissolved in blood also has a partial pressure. The amount of gas capable of dissolving in blood depends on its solubility and partial pressure. Gases always move from higher to lower pressure.[3]
   3. The rate at which gases are exchanged depends primarily on the difference between partial pressures. If the gas entering the alveolus has a significantly higher partial pressure than that in the capillary, the gas rapidly diffuses into the blood. This occurs until the partial pressure in the blood equals that of the alveoli.
       a. When N_2O/O_2 is administered, high concentrations of these gases are found in the alveolus, creating a high partial pressure. The capillary, possessing no N_2O originally, is quickly filled.
       b. N_2O is not readily absorbed by the blood. Because of this insolubility, very little gas is absorbed into blood elements. Within minutes, equilibrium between the partial pressures of the alveolus and capillary is achieved. This quick action continues as the N_2O is carried to the brain; the onset of clinical effect is rapid once the gas reaches the brain.
       c. The converse of rapid infusion to the blood is also true. As the N_2O flow is terminated, capillary tension quickly rises to that above alveolar pressure. N_2O is quickly forced into the alveoli and exhaled through the lungs. Trace amounts of N_2O are metabolized in the body; however, most is removed rapidly through the lungs. During this process, N_2O exits faster than the N_2 that replaces it, thereby diluting the supply of O_2 and reducing the O_2 blood saturation (SaO_2). This phenomenon is called diffusion hypoxia.

F. Pulse oximetry provides determination of O_2 saturation of arterial blood. O_2 saturation refers to the amount of O_2 carried by the hemoglobin.
   1. In a healthy patient with no pulmonary or cardiovascular disease, O_2 saturation should be between 98% and 100%.[4] There are certain factors that can affect this value. Such factors include altitude (e.g., Denver, Colorado, USA at 5280 feet). Local factors such as nail polish can affect the measurement of this value.
   2. The pulse oximeter operates on the principle that hemoglobin exists in two forms in the blood, either oxygenated in arterial blood with O_2 molecules loosely bound (HbO_2) or reduced hemoglobin with no O_2 molecules bound (Hb). The amount of arterial saturation (SpO_2) is the ratio of oxygenated hemoglobin to the total. The pulse oximeter

---

Box 8-1   **COMPOSITION OF AMBIENT AIR**

20.94% oxygen (O_2)
79.02% nitrogen (N_2)
0.04% carbon dioxide (CO_2)

measures the absorption of selected wavelengths of light as they pass through living tissue. A sensor is most commonly applied to the fingertip (Figures 8-6 and 8-7). HbO_2 and Hb absorb these wavelengths of light to different extents. The amount of O_2 saturation of arterial blood (SpO_2) as a percentage is displayed on the pulse oximeter screen. Pulse oximeters frequently monitor heart rate and may even include blood pressure values as well.

3. It is important to recognize that any O_2 saturation level less than 90% is a matter of grave concern and is a clear early warning of impending rapid loss of O_2 to the brain.

4. *Although use of a pulse oximeter is not mandated to monitor O_2 saturation for minimal sedation, it is required for moderate sedation according to the ASA Practice Guidelines for Non-Anesthesiologists.* Therefore, it can be useful in detecting potential early problems with N_2O/O_2 administration should the line between minimal and moderate sedation (50% N_2O concentration) be crossed. The AAP/AAPD guidelines suggest the use of a pulse oximeter that uses auditory tones when changes in hemoglobin saturation occur.[5]

G. Diffusion hypoxia

1. It has been hypothesized that headache, lethargy, and nausea can occur because of decreased O_2 saturation levels in the blood caused by the rapid exit of N_2O on its termination. The application of 100% pure O_2 for the first 3–5 minutes after N_2O termination has been traditionally advocated to prevent O_2 desaturation of blood. Jeske *et al*[6] disagree with this practice and report no diffusion hypoxia when breathing room air instead of 100% O_2.

2. Researchers question the clinical significance of diffusion hypoxia and whether these symptoms are even associated. Quarnstrom *et al*[7] evaluated 104 patients and found no drop in SaO_2. They question the necessity for postoperative O_2. Papageorge *et al*[8] monitored 80 patients and found O_2 decreased with a mean of 2.1%. In this study, all O_2 decreases stabilized independently within 12 seconds to 15 minutes. Dunn-Russell *et al*[9] assessed 24 children who were allowed to breathe room air after N_2O/O_2 sedation. None exhibited abnormal SaO_2 levels or exhibited any of the associated side

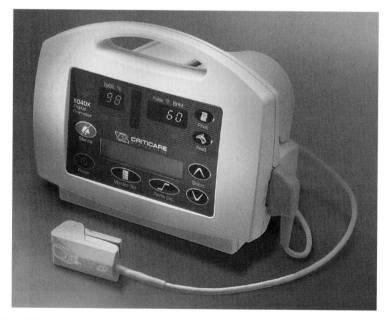

Figure 8-6 Pulse oximeter with digital sensor. *(Courtesy Criticare Systems, Inc., Waukesha, Wisconsin.)*

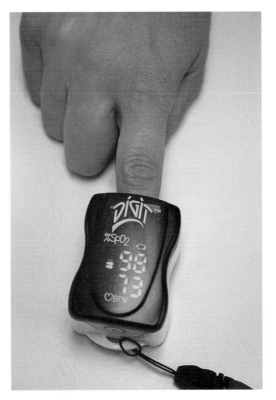

Figure 8-7 Digital sensor attached to finger.

effects. Murphy and Splinter[10] claimed the same conclusion with children undergoing general anesthesia. Brodsky *et al*[11] observed only 3 of 60 patients with SaO_2 decreases. Hovagim *et al*[12] state that even when postoperative O_2 is given, there may be mild decreases in O_2 saturation. Leelataweewud *et al*[13] stated no differences in SpO_2 or pulse rate when pediatric subjects were given N_2O or O_2 the SpO_2 readings remained near 97% throughout the study.

3. Although researchers claim diffusion hypoxia is not clinically significant, some patients experience postoperative headache, lethargy, and nausea when 100% postoperative O_2 is not given. Administering 100% O_2 postoperatively for a minimum of 5 minutes prevents these symptoms from occurring. Lampe *et al*[14] agree that it continues to be prudent practice to deliver O_2 postoperatively. As authors, we concur that postoperative O_2 should be given at a minimum of 5 minutes and until the patient recovers.

VI. MANAGEMENT OF PATIENTS EXPERIENCING MODERATE SEDATION (LEVELS OF N_2O GREATER THAN 50%)

A. Guidelines. Nonanesthesiologists who treat patients in a hospital setting are legally required to adhere to the ASA practice guidelines previously referenced. Private practitioners, although not required to follow these guidelines, should seriously consider the use of these standards in their offices, because the guidelines describe the standards of care that have been established by the practitioners' hospital-based peers. Again, the practitioner is responsible for the possible complications associated with the intended level of sedation and those associated with the next (deeper) level. Therefore, because moderate sedation may occur or be intended, considerations for obstructed airway and preprocedure fasting guidelines are addressed.

VII. AIRWAY MANAGEMENT

A. Airway obstruction in the upper airway represents an acute life-threatening situation.[15]
   1. This is commonly the result of the dorsum of the tongue occluding with the posterior pharyngeal wall. Another common cause of airway obstruction is the presence of a foreign body.[16]
   2. During moderate sedation, the laryngeal and pharyngeal reflexes should remain intact at all times, thereby allowing the cough and gag reflexes to protect the airway.

B. The universal distress signal for choking is to grasp the throat with both hands.
   1. If a foreign body airway obstruction is suspected in a conscious individual, ask the person "Are you choking?"
   2. Apply the Heimlich maneuver until the foreign object is expelled or the person becomes unconscious.
   3. Summon emergency personnel immediately for any unconscious person. Perform chest thrusts and attempt to ventilate the lungs similar to cardiopulmonary resuscitation (CPR) until medical assistance arrives.[17]

C. A simple hyperextension (head tilt–chin lift) or jaw thrust maneuver should relieve an airway obstruction that is not caused by the presence of a foreign body.
   1. A partial airway obstruction will allow the patient to make sounds. A snoring sound can indicate a partial airway obstruction caused by the posterior displacement of the tongue.[16]
   2. With a complete airway obstruction, no sound occurs.
   3. A full-face mask replacing the nasal hood and a reservoir bag filled with oxygen can provide positive pressurized oxygen into the lungs, making the sedation unit an excellent piece of emergency management equipment.

D. The pulse oximeter should be left in place at all times to continuously monitor oxygen saturation.

E. Aspiration of vomitus is unlikely when the protective airway reflexes are intact.
   1. Should vomiting occur, the patient should be placed in an upright position and vomitus cleared from the oral cavity.
   2. The pharynx should be suctioned to remove any vomitus. O_2 should be administered, and the patient should be evaluated for the possibility of any aspiration.[16]

VIII. PREPROCEDURAL FASTING GUIDELINES

A. Preprocedure fasting guidelines are recommended in the ASA practice guidelines. These guidelines are to be used when moderate sedation is achieved intentionally or unintentionally. It is recommended that a light meal with no fried or fatty foods be consumed at least 6 hours before sedation procedures and that no liquids be consumed within 2 hours of the procedure. A complete summary of the ASA preprocedure fasting guidelines may be found in Chapter 10.

REFERENCES

1. Light RW: Mechanics of respiration. In George RB *et al*, editors: *Chest Medicine: Essentials of Pulmonary and Critical Care Medicine*, Baltimore, 1995, Williams & Wilkins.
2. George RB, Chesson AL, Rennard SI: Functional anatomy of the respiratory system. In George RB *et al*, editors: *Chest Medicine: Essentials of Pulmonary and Critical Care Medicine*, Baltimore, 1995, Williams & Wilkins.
3. Stoelting RD: *Pharmacology and Physiology in Anesthetic Practice*, ed 2, Philadelphia, 1991, JB Lippincott.
4. Shapiro BA: *Oxygenation: Measurement and Clinical Assessment*, Philadelphia, 1979, JB Lippincott.
5. AAP/AAPD Clinical Report: Guidelines for monitoring and management of pediatric patients during and after sedation for diagnostic and therapeutic procedures: an update, *Pediatrics* 118(6):2587, December 2006.
6. Jeske AH *et al*: Noninvasive assessment of diffusion hypoxia following administration of nitrous oxide-oxygen, *Anesth Prog* 51(1):10, 2004.
7. Quarnstrom FC *et al*: Clinical study of diffusion hypoxia after nitrous oxide analgesia, *Anesth Prog* 38:21, 1991.
8. Papageorge, MB, Noonan LW Jr, Rosenberg M: Diffusion hypoxia: another view, *Anesth Pain Control Dent* 2:143, 1993.
9. Dunn-Russell T *et al*: Oxygen saturation and diffusion hypoxia in children following nitrous oxide sedation, *Pediatr Dent* 16:88, 1993.
10. Murphy IL, Splinter WM: The clinical significance of diffusion hypoxia in children, *Can J Anaesth* 37:S40, 1990.
11. Brodsky JB *et al*: Diffusion hypoxia: a reappraisal using pulse oximetry, *J Clin Mon* 4:244, 1988.
12. Hovagim AR *et al*: Arterial oxygen desaturation in adult dental patients receiving conscious sedation, *J Oral Maxillofac Surg* 47:936, 1989.
13. Leelataweewud P *et al*: The physiological effects of supplemental oxygen versus nitrous oxide/oxygen during conscious sedation of pediatric dental patients, *Pediatr Dent* 22(2):125, 2000.
14. Lampe GH *et al*: Postoperative hypoxemia after nonabdominal surgery: a frequent event not caused by nitrous oxide, *Anesth Analg* 71:597, 1990.
15. Malamed SF: *Medical Emergencies in the Dental Office*, ed 6, St. Louis, 2007, Mosby.
16. Malamed SF: *Sedation: A Guide to Patient Management*, ed 4, St. Louis, 2003, Mosby.
17. American Heart Association: Guidelines 2000 for CPR and emergency cardiovascular care, *Curr Emerg Cardiovasc Care* 11(3):11, 2000.

SUGGESTED READINGS

Artru AA: Survival time during hypoxia: effects of nitrous oxide, thiopental, and hypothermia, *Anesth Analg* 67:913, 1988.

Eger EI II: Respiratory effects of nitrous oxide. In Eger EI II: *Nitrous Oxide N_2O*, New York, 1985, Elsevier Science Publishing.

Mueller WA *et al*: Pulse oximetry monitoring of sedated pediatric dental patients, *Anesth Prog* 32:237, 1985.

Papageorge MB *et al*: Supplemental oxygen after outpatient oral and maxillofacial surgery, *Anesth Prog* 39:24, 1993.

N₂O and Its Interactions with the Body

Nitrous oxide has been in continuous use as an anxiolytic drug because it is a safe drug. It is compatible with human physiology, and when administered with oxygen, it actually improves a patient's perfusion while decreasing his or her anxiety. This chapter will explore how nitrous oxide interacts with the specific body systems. In addition, basic knowledge of nitrous oxide is important to keep one aware of potential interactions with new drugs sure to find their way into the marketplace. Although every drug has some impact on the human physiology, nitrous oxide is eliminated very rapidly and very completely back through the lungs, whereas an infinitesimal amount is excreted in urine and sweat glands. This rapid elimination further indicates the temporary nature of the drug. Therefore, in today's world of increasing human longevity, nitrous oxide finds its use across the spectrum from pediatric to geriatric and the healthy to the medically compromised.

I. N₂O INTERACTION WITH BODY SYSTEMS AND CONDITIONS

A. Cardiovascular system

1. N_2O does not negatively affect the cardiovascular system to produce any significant physiologic changes. The interaction of several cardiovascular functions, such as contractility, output, stroke volume, heart rate, and arrhythmias, with N_2O have been researched in the past.[1-5] Overall, N_2O has proven to be slightly cardiotonic.

2. N_2O effects on cardiac output differ in the literature. Slight increases have been noted, as well as mild decreases. Dosage and the sympathomimetic effects of the drug may account for subtle differences.[1-5]

3. Blood flow to major organs is not significantly affected.[3]

4. N_2O with O_2 does not create adverse cardiovascular conditions. Conversely, it has a positive effect on myocardial ischemia by providing supplemental O_2 and can be very helpful in myocardial infarction.[6,7]

5. Blood pressure effects from N_2O may be dose related. In most instances, blood pressure is not affected by the N_2O concentrations commonly used in ambulatory settings. Eger *et al*[1] found blood pressure readings to be lowered when N_2O/O_2 was used. This potential decrease in blood pressure is a result of relaxation, because N_2O does not have any direct effect on the myocardium or voluntary skeletal muscle.

6. Nitrous oxide has a minimal effect on heart rate.[8] As with blood pressure, heart rate may decrease as anxiety is lowered.

◆ N₂O/O₂ Use Indicated in Ambulatory Setting

Atherosclerosis or arteriosclerosis
Rheumatic fever, heart murmur, congenital conditions
Angina pectoris, myocardial infarction

Surgery (valve, pacemaker, bypass, transplant)
Hypertension

⑥ N$_2$O/O$_2$ Use Considered/Medical Consultation Advised

No conditions known at this time

⚠ N$_2$O/O$_2$ Use Contraindicated or Postponed Until Condition Resolved

No conditions known at this time

B. **Respiratory system**
1. Upper respiratory tract infections or conditions commonly compromise air exchange through the nose. If the patient is unable to breathe through the nose, insufficient amounts of N$_2$O/O$_2$ will enter the respiratory system.
    a. Any type of common infection leading to a cold, cough, sinus infection, bronchitis, allergy-related symptoms, etc. may occlude the nasal passages such that adequate air exchange at the alveolar level will be incomplete.
    b. In addition, if N$_2$O/O$_2$ is used for an individual with mild symptoms, the drying effect of the gases may create mucous plugs and negatively affect the pulmonary tree. Again, sedation may be incomplete and inadequate.
    c. Sinus cavities represent rigid, noncompliant air spaces. The nonexpansive nature of these areas leads to an increase in pressure when N$_2$O is administered. When sinusitis is present, the additional pressure may be uncomfortable for the patient.
2. Although rare, silent regurgitation and subsequent aspiration need to be considered with N$_2$O/O$_2$ sedation. The concern lies in whether pharyngeal-laryngeal reflexes remain intact. This problem can be avoided by not allowing a patient to go into an unconscious state.[9]
    a. Dye studies done with a 5- to 10-minute exposure to 50% N$_2$O were negative for aspiration[10]; no evidence of aspiration occurred in 25 children given N$_2$O concentrations between 20% and 65%.[11]
    b. Procedures performed in an ambulatory health setting may or may not be time intensive; however, patients may not have fasted before the procedure. Therefore, the potential for positive aspiration resulting from silent regurgitation does exist.
    c. Because this is a potentially life-threatening situation, it is important to use the appropriate titration technique when administering N$_2$O/O$_2$ sedation to avoid oversedation. Continuous monitoring of the patient should always be carried out.
3. Patients susceptible to hypoxia because of airway resistance, impaired function, or movement seem to be at a slight risk from N$_2$O/O$_2$ sedation but not more than any other substances. Examples of conditions in this category are emphysema and chronic bronchitis.
    a. There has never been a reported allergy to N$_2$O. Its use is not contraindicated for asthma patients, because it is nonirritating to mucous membranes. In fact, the sedative nature of N$_2$O/O$_2$ has a positive influence on asthmatic patients, as anxiety can trigger an asthmatic episode.
    b. For patients chronically debilitated with other respiratory conditions, N$_2$O/O$_2$ may be considered relatively contraindicated (Box 9-1).
        i. Some of these patients may be on hypoxic drive. Although CO$_2$ normally initiates respiration in healthy individuals, O$_2$ may be the stimulus for those compromised with chronic obstructive pulmonary diseases (COPD).

Box 9-1 | **RELATIVE CONTRAINDICATIONS FOR USE OF N₂O/O₂ SEDATION**

- First trimester of pregnancy
- Pneumothorax
- Cystic fibrosis
- Current upper respiratory tract infection
- Chronic obstructive pulmonary diseases
- Psychologic impairment
- Current or recovering drug use/addiction
- Middle ear disturbance/surgery (i.e., grafting)
- Bleomycin therapy
- Inability to understand procedure
- Phobic individuals
- Current psychotropic drug use
- Recent pneumoencephalography

---

      ii.   Patients with severe chronic respiratory diseases should receive medical consultation before undergoing any type of sedation. Any kind of sedation may risk further depression of their respiratory drive.

      iii.   In most cases, persons on hypoxic drive are very ill. Some will not be able to be treated in an ambulatory setting; most represent an ASA III or IV classification (see Chapter 10). Medical consultation is recommended before any treatment.

   4.   Patients with cystic fibrosis may incur bullae as a complication of this disease, again because of the expansive nature of the gas. N_2O would be contraindicated in this case.[12]

   5.   The condition of pneumothorax (air or gas in the pleural cavity) may be complicated with N_2O. The expansive quality of the gas causes increased expansion of the size of the pneumothorax. This condition demands medical attention. In general anesthesia, if 75% N_2O is delivered, the volume of the space can be increased up to 300%.[13] Although in the ambulatory setting the doses of N_2O are much smaller, the pharmacodynamic nature of the gas is constant. N_2O/O_2 sedation should be avoided in this situation.

▶ N₂O/O₂ Use Indicated (in Ambulatory Setting)

Asthma

◎ N₂O/O₂ Use Considered/Medical Consultation Advised

Emphysema
Chronic bronchitis

▽ N₂O/O₂ Use Contraindicated or Postponed Until Condition Resolved

Upper respiratory tract infections
Pneumothorax
Cystic fibrosis

C. **Central nervous system (CNS)**
   1. N_2O, like other anesthetics, has the ability to depress the CNS; however, the exact mechanism is unknown.[4]
   2. N_2O's effects on cerebral blood flow, intracranial pressure, cerebral blood velocity, cerebral perfusion pressure, and O_2 consumption have been compared with other

anesthetics.[14,15] Most effects seem to be less significant than that of other inhaled anesthetics.[4,16] When nitrous oxide is used appropriately with oxygen in the ambulatory setting, these effects are not significant.

3. The dosage of N$_2$O has an effect on the frequency and voltage changes on electroencephalograms (EEGs).[4,16]

4. Because of the rapid replacement of N$_2$ with N$_2$O in air spaces, notable intracranial pressure increases were found in cases of pneumoencephalography. N$_2$O should not be used for 1 week after this procedure.[16]

5. Evidence of injury to the nervous system has been shown in cases of chronic exposure to N$_2$O. Numbness and weakness in the extremities are seen as symptoms, as is ataxic gait.[2] This subject is discussed in detail in Chapter 17.

N$_2$O/O$_2$ Use Indicated in Ambulatory Setting

Cerebrovascular accident (stroke)
Seizure disorder
Parkinson's disease, etc.

N$_2$O/O$_2$ Use Considered/Medical Consultation Advised

No conditions known at this time

N$_2$O/O$_2$ Use Contraindicated or Postponed Until Condition Resolved

Recent pneumoencephalography
Known nitrous oxide abuse

D. **Hematopoietic system**

1. Megaloblastic bone marrow changes have been found in patients who have been exposed to high concentrations of N$_2$O for an extended period.[17] N$_2$O has been implicated in the interference of the vitamin B$_{12}$–dependent enzyme methionine synthase for many years. This enzyme is necessary for DNA synthesis and erythrocyte production.[4,16] Research continues regarding hematological effects and nitrous oxide. The current issue raised is in individuals who are vitamin B$_{12}$ deficient.[8,18] Pernicious anemia and megaloblastic anemia are conditions that are associated with this vitamin deficiency, and malabsorption is the primary cause of this deficiency. In addition, a correlation exists between an imbalanced vitamin B$_{12}$ metabolism and increased homocysteine levels. The studies citing hematologic effects associated with nitrous oxide are those when nitrous oxide is used as an anesthetic where doses are high and events are time intensive.[4,18,19] The literature has not cited significant effects with low-dose nitrous oxide exposures for minimal periods of time.[17]

2. Another concern with hematopoietic conditions is the decrease in O$_2$ available to the body because of red blood cell deficiency, impairment, destruction, and/or other conditions affecting red blood cells. Inhalation sedation can be recommended because of the supplemental O$_2$ it delivers.[20]

N$_2$O/O$_2$ Use Indicated in Ambulatory Setting

Anemias
Methemoglobinemia
Sickle cell anemia
Leukemia
Hemophilia
Polycythemia vera

⊚ **N$_2$0/O$_2$ Use Considered/Medical Consultation Advised**

No conditions known at this time

▽ **N$_2$0/O$_2$ Use Contraindicated or Postponed Until Condition Resolved**

No conditions known at this time

E. **Endocrine system**
    1. Inhalation sedation with N_2O/O_2 has no negative effect on the endocrine system.

◆ **N$_2$0/O$_2$ Use Indicated in Ambulatory Setting**

Diabetes
Thyroid gland dysfunction
Adrenal dysfunction

⊚ **N$_2$0/O$_2$ Use Considered/Medical Consultation Advised**

No conditions known at this time

▽ **N$_2$0/O$_2$ Use Contraindicated or Postponed Until Condition Resolved**

No conditions known at this time

F. **Hepatic system**
    1. N_2O is not metabolized in the liver, nor does it affect the liver in the presence of liver impairment.[1,21–23]

◆ **N$_2$0/O$_2$ Use Indicated in Ambulatory Setting**

Hepatitis
Jaundice
Cirrhosis

⊚ **N$_2$0/O$_2$ Use Considered/Medical Consultation Advised**

No conditions known at this time

▽ **N$_2$0/O$_2$ Use Contraindicated or Postponed Until Condition Resolved**

No conditions known at this time

G. **Gastrointestinal system**
    1. Because of the expansive nature of the gas and its propensity for insufflating air spaces within the body, N_2O diffuses into these areas much more rapidly than N_2 exits. The gas entering nonrigid-walled air spaces in the body causes the spaces to expand. This expansion and possible pressure can be problematic.
    2. The bowel exemplifies a nonrigid air space in which expansion occurs. If a patient has a bowel obstruction, it is less desirable to use N_2O/O_2 sedation, because the N_2O can affect the condition by increasing expansion, pressure, and discomfort.[24]

◆ **N$_2$0/O$_2$ Use Indicated in Ambulatory Setting**

Ulcer
Gastroesophageal reflux disorder (GERD)

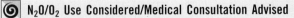 **N₂0/0₂ Use Considered/Medical Consultation Advised**

No conditions known at this time

N₂0/0₂ Use Contraindicated or Postponed Until Condition Resolved

Bowel obstruction

H. Genitourinary and reproductive systems

1. N_2O/O_2 sedation does not pose any negative effect on the genitourinary system itself. Any time disease transmissibility is an issue, proper infection control procedures and sterilization of appropriate equipment is recommended.

2. Pregnancy is a normal physiologic state that requires twice the demand for folate. Treatment considerations are important during organogenesis in the first trimester and when low O_2 tension levels are possible in the last trimester. Most pharmacologic agents cross the placental barrier; N_2O is no exception.

   a. It is necessary to maintain adequate O_2 levels to prevent spontaneous abortion. However, the O_2 fail-safe feature incorporated in newer equipment prevents this occurrence.

   b. The N_2O/O_2 combination has been a commonly used pharmacologic agent in obstetrics. Research confirms its safety with pregnant women.[25] In case of pregnancy, the following items regarding N_2O/O_2 sedation in the ambulatory setting should be considered:

      i. Obtain appropriate medical consultation before the use of any drug for the duration of the pregnancy.

      ii. Avoid N_2O during the first trimester. N_2O, when delivered appropriately, should not physiologically threaten the fetus; however, like radiation, N_2O/O_2 could be blamed unfairly should fetal anomalies occur.

      iii. It is best to leave the decision whether to use N_2O/O_2 sedation to the patient and attending medical personnel.

N₂0/0₂ Use Indicated (in Ambulatory Setting)

Kidney disease
Sexually transmitted diseases

N₂0/0₂ Use Considered/Medical Consultation Advised

Pregnancy

N₂0/0₂ Use Contraindicated or Postponed Until Condition Resolved

Pregnancy

I. Neuromuscular system

1. N_2O does not provide direct skeletal muscle relaxation, but it does so indirectly. In high concentrations, muscle rigidity can be seen with N_2O secondary to anxiety.[26] However, Yoshida presented a reduction in orofacial muscle tone during dental treatment with nitrous oxide in patients with cerebral palsy.[27]

2. N_2O/O_2 has no effect on patients with neuromuscular conditions.

N₂0/0₂ Use Indicated (in Ambulatory Setting)

Multiple sclerosis
Muscular dystrophy

Cerebral palsy
Myasthenia gravis
Other

⊚ **N₂O/O₂ Use Considered/Medical Consultation Advised**

No conditions known at this time

⚠ **N₂O/O₂ Use Contraindicated or Postponed Until Condition Resolved**

No conditions known at this time

J. **Cancer**
    1. N_2O does not combine with any of the formed blood elements, nor does it affect metastatic cells.[20]
    2. N_2O/O_2 has been used in the final stages of life as an adjuvant to other pharmacologic methods for pain and anxiety management. In these situations the untoward effects caused by chronic exposure to N_2O are irrelevant.[28,29]
    3. Patients currently receiving bleomycin sulfate, an antineoplastic agent used typically for the treatment of lymphomas, testicular tumors, and squamous cell carcinomas, can increase the incidence of pulmonary fibrosis and other pulmonary disease. This occurs only indirectly if O_2 is administered concomitantly with N_2O in concentrations greater than 30%. Although this is an unusual situation, it must be regarded.[30]

◆ **N₂O/O₂ Use Indicated (in Ambulatory Setting)**

Cancer

⊚ **N₂O/O₂ Use Considered/Medical Consultation Advised**

No conditions known at this time

⚠ **N₂O/O₂ Use Contraindicated or Postponed Until Condition Resolved**

Bleomycin sulfate therapy

K. **Allergies**
    1. For more than 160 years, there have been no known reported allergies to N_2O.
    2. Persons sensitive to latex may experience contact dermatitis when using a nasal hood made from rubber products. Latex-free nasal hoods, conduction tubing, and reservoir bags are available from and exclusively produced by each equipment manufacturer in the United States.

◆ **N₂O/O₂ Use Indicated (in Ambulatory Setting)**

Allergies—use latex-free products

⊚ **N₂O/O₂ Use Considered/Medical Consultation Advised**

No conditions known at this time

⚠ **N₂O/O₂ Use Contraindicated or Postponed Until Condition Resolved**

No conditions known at this time

L. **Malignant hyperthermia (MH)**
    1. This condition may unexpectedly occur as a result of an individual's response to certain drugs. Patients who know of familial tendencies and history can be tested to avoid this problem.

2. N$_2$O/O$_2$ sedation is not considered a trigger for malignant hyperthermia and can be safely administered to MH-susceptible individuals.[8]

M. Nutritional disorders

1. N$_2$O/O$_2$ sedation does not affect any nutritional condition. Research is ongoing in this area.

N. Mind-altering conditions

1. Mind-altering conditions indicate situations warranting careful consideration before N$_2$O/O$_2$ administration, because nitrous oxide itself is a substance that produces euphoria. Patients should be able to understand the procedure and its effects, or otherwise they may negatively perceive the associated signs and symptoms of N$_2$O/O$_2$ sedation.

   a. For patients with a mental deficiency such as Down syndrome, it is necessary to determine the ability of the individual to understand the sedation procedure. If the patient can understand what to expect and is able to distinguish if or when he or she would become uncomfortable, then it would be appropriate to administer nitrous oxide and oxygen. If that level of understanding is not present or the practitioner is unable to determine it, nitrous oxide and oxygen should not be used. The same rationale is used for persons with Alzheimer's disease or autism. This type of sedation can be used as long as the level of understanding is present and there are not other conditions present that would be relative contraindications.[31,32]

2. N$_2$O/O$_2$ use should be avoided for a patient intoxicated with drugs or alcohol. Although alcohol is initially a stimulant, it has been historically prescribed and acknowledged as a mild anxiolytic over time. It should never be present when a healthcare provider is administering N$_2$O and O$_2$. Alcohol and barbiturates are potent CNS depressants.

3. Barbiturates are quite effective sedative agents when prescribed in therapeutic doses; however, patients prescribing their own drugs and dosages before their appointments should not be treated.

4. If the patient is suffering or recovering from addiction or mental illness, the relaxing, euphoric sensations from nitrous oxide may exacerbate or trigger unwanted episodes or may encourage addictive behaviors. Discretion is warranted.

5. Patients under psychiatric and/or psychological care should be carefully considered before N$_2$O/O$_2$ use. Many patients are treated with antidepressant or other psychotropic drugs. It is important to understand the pharmacology of these drugs and be aware of any synergistic effects. Seek medical consultation before N$_2$O/O$_2$ administration.

6. N$_2$O may enhance drugs that are used directly to induce sleep or that list drowsiness as a side effect. Again, seek medical consultation to determine the extent of the underlying condition. Ensure that the patient has not just recently taken these drugs before N$_2$O/O$_2$ administration.

7. Severely phobic individuals will not benefit by N$_2$O/O$_2$ administration. These persons should be in the care of a competent expert in behavior management. It is unlikely that N$_2$O/O$_2$ will be able to provide adequate relief to accomplish the intended procedure. It is likely that N$_2$O/O$_2$ will make the situation worse, because the patient will resist the calming effects of the drug. Physical agitation and acts of aggression can result. Deep sedation or general anesthesia will, most likely, be the procedure of choice in this situation.

8. In some cases, patients with claustrophobic tendencies may feel uncomfortable with the use of a nasal hood. Often these patients relax sufficiently during N$_2$O/O$_2$ sedation that this is not a problem.

N$_2$O/O$_2$ Use Indicated (In Ambulatory Setting)

As advised in following categories

◉ N₂O/O₂ Use Considered/Medical Consultation Advised

Mind-altering conditions
Recovering alcohol or drug addiction
Patients taking antidepressant or psychotropic drugs
Patient who has taken medication to induce sleep

▽! N₂O/O₂ Use Contraindicated or Postponed Until Condition Resolved

Mind-altering conditions
Current chemical dependency including alcoholism and substance abuse
Patients taking antidepressant or psychotropic drugs
Patient who has taken medication to induce sleep
Phobias, including claustrophobia

O. **Other**
   1. Middle ear disturbances
      a. Because N_2O infiltrates the rigid, noncompliant area of the middle ear, increased pressure results. Complications have been noted with middle ear surgical procedures with N_2O.[33] Significant damage such as tympanic membrane rupture, graft displacement, and other complications have been observed.[33–38] Also, the negative pressure that results from the rapid departure of N_2O after general anesthesia can cause other side effects, especially after recent ear, nose, and throat complications.[39] The conditions just listed refer to surgical procedures that use anesthetic concentrations of N_2O. There is no mention whether these complications occur with lower concentrations used in minimal sedation.
   2. Eye surgery
      a. A safety alert was published about patients and recent ophthalmic surgery in which perfluoropropane or sulfur hexafluoride gas was used. In patients undergoing vitreoretinal procedures, typically, a "gas bubble" is placed in the eye to assist the healing process; this gas bubble could expand with N_2O and complicate healing or promote injury.[40]
      b. Patients should be questioned about recent ophthalmic surgery before N_2O/O_2 sedation is used.[41]
   3. For those professionals in emergency medicine, whether in the field or hospital, it is unwise to use N_2O/O_2 for anyone in shock, in a semiconscious state, or with head or facial injuries.
   4. When time is taken to explain the N_2O/O_2 procedure and words are carefully chosen to present the positive effects of the gas, most patients will consent and do well. If a patient is unwilling or does not give consent, the practitioner must never force the continuance of the procedure. This may destroy any patient-operator trust and place the practitioner in legal jeopardy.

⬌ N₂O/O₂ Use Indicated (in Ambulatory Setting)

As advised in categories below

◉ N₂O/O₂ Use Considered/Medical Consultation Advised

Recent tympanic membrane graft
Recent eye surgery with perfluoropropane or sulfur hexafluoride gas

▽! N₂O/O₂ Use Contraindicated or Postponed until Condition Resolved

Recent tympanic membrane graft
Recent eye surgery with perfluoropropane or sulfur hexafluoride gas
Patient in shock, semiconscious state, head or facial injuries
Unwilling patient or one who does not consent

REFERENCES

1. Eger EI II, *et al*: Clinical pharmacology of nitrous oxide: an argument for its continued use, *Anesth Anal* 71:575, 1990.
2. Eger EI II, Gaskey NJ: A review of the present status of nitrous oxide, *J Assoc Nurse Anes* 54:29, 1986.
3. Eisele JH, Jr: Cardiovascular effects of nitrous oxide. In Eger EI II, editor: *Nitrous Oxide N₂O*, New York, 1985, Elsevier Science Publishing.
4. Stoelting RK: *Pharmacology and Physiology in Anesthetic Practice*, ed 2, Philadelphia, 1991, JB Lippincott.
5. Stoelting RK, Miller RD: *Basics of Anesthesia*, ed 2, New York, 1989, Churchill Livingstone.
6. Thompson PL, Lown B: Nitrous oxide as an analgesic in acute myocardial infarction, *JAMA* 235:924, 1976.
7. Kerr F *et al*: Nitrous oxide analgesia in myocardial infarction, *Lancet* 1:63, 1972.
8. Eger E: Current status of nitrous oxide, Unpublished research, 2006.
9. Eger EI II: Respiratory effects of nitrous oxide. In Eger EI II, editor: *Nitrous Oxide N₂O*, New York, 1985, Elsevier Science Publishing.
10. Cleaton-Jones P: The laryngeal-closure reflex and nitrous oxide-oxygen anesthesia, *Anesthesiology* 45:569, 1976.
11. Roberts GJ, Wignall BK: Efficacy of the laryngeal reflex during oxygen-nitrous oxide sedation (relative analgesia), *Br J Anesth* 54:1277, 1982.
12. Goodman BE, Percy WH: CFTR in cystic fibrosis and cholera: from membrane transport to clinical practice, *Advan Physiol Edu* 29:75, 2005.
13. Eger EI II, Saidman LJ: Hazards of nitrous oxide anesthesia in bowel obstruction and pneumothorax, *Anesthesiology* 26:61, 1965.
14. Hancock SM, Eastwood JR, Mahajan RP: Effects of inhaled nitrous oxide 50% on estimated cerebral perfusion pressure and zero flow pressure in healthy volunteers, *Anaesthesia* 60:129, 2005.
15. Mathew RJ, *et al*: Effect of nitrous oxide on cerebral blood velocity while reclining and standing, *Biol Psychiatry* 41:979, 1997.
16. Frost EA: Central nervous system effects of nitrous oxide. In Eger EI II, editor: *Nitrous Oxide N₂O*, New York, 1985, Elsevier Science Publishing.
17. Nunn JE: Clinical aspects of the interaction between nitrous oxide and vitamin B_{12}, *Br J Anesth* 59:3, 1987.
18. Weimann J: Toxicity of nitrous oxide, *Best Pract Res Clin Anaesthesiol* 17(1):47, 2003.
19. Myles PS *et al*: A review of the risks and benefits of nitrous oxide in current anaesthetic practice, *Anaesth Intensive Care* 32:165, 2004.
20. Malamed SF: *Sedation: A Guide to Patient Management*, ed 4, St. Louis, 2003, Mosby.
21. Brodsky JB: Toxicity of nitrous oxide. In Eger EI II, editor: *Nitrous Oxide N₂O*, New York, 1985, Elsevier Science Publishing.
22. Lampe GJ *et al*: Nitrous oxide does not impair hepatic function on young or old surgical patients, *Anesth Analg* 71:606, 1990.
23. Longnecker DE, Miller FL: Pharmacology of inhalation anesthetics. In Rogers M *et al*, editors: *Principles and Practice of Anesthesiology*, St. Louis, 1993, Mosby.
24. Eger EI II: Pharmacokinetics. In Eger EI II, editor: *Nitrous Oxide N₂O*, New York, 1985, Elsevier Science Publishing.
25. Marx FG, Bassell GM: Nitrous oxide in obsterics. In Eger EI II, editor: *Nitrous Oxide N₂O*, New York, 1985, Elsevier Science Publishing.
26. Miller RD: Neuromuscular effects of nitrous oxide. In Eger EI II, editor: *Nitrous Oxide N₂O*, New York, 1985, Elsevier Science Publishing.
27. Yoshida M *et al*: Effect of nitrous oxide on dental patients with cerebral palsy—using an electromyogram (EMG) from orofacial muscles as an index, *J Oral Rehab* 30:324, 2003.
28. Fosburg MT, Crone RK: Nitrous oxide analgesia for refractory pain in the terminally ill, *JAMA* 250:511, 1983.
29. Foley LM: The treatment of pain in the patient with cancer, *CA Cancer J Clin* 36:194, 1986.
30. Fleming P, Walker PO, Priest JR: Bleomycin therapy: a contraindication to the use of nitrous oxide-oxygen psychosedation in the dental office, *Pediatr Dent* 10(4):345, 1988.
31. Friedlander AH *et al*: The neuropathology, medical management and dental implications of autism, *JADA* 137:1517, 2006.
32. Dental Anesthesia for the Austistic Child, Autism Research Institute, *http://autism.com*, 2006.
33. Munson ES: Complications of nitrous oxide anesthesia for ear surgery, *Anesthesiology* 11(3):559, 1993.
34. Donlon JV, Jr: Anesthesia and eye, ear, nose, and throat surgery. In Miller RD: *Anesthesia*, ed 4, New York, 1994, Churchill Livingstone.
35. Barash P, Cullen B, Stoelting R: *Clinical Anesthesia*, ed 2, Philadelphia, 1992, JB Lippincott.

36. Mann MS, Woodsford PV, Jones RM: Anesthetic carrier gases, *Anesthesiology* 40:8, 1985.
37. Waun JE, Sweitzer RH, Hamilton WK: Effect of nitrous oxide on middle ear mechanics and hearing activity, *Anesthesiology* 28:846, 1967.
38. Ohryn M: Tympanic membrane rupture following general anesthesia with nitrous oxide: a case report, *J Am Assoc Nurse Anesth* 63:42, 1995.
39. Chinn K *et al*: Middle ear pressure variation: effect of nitrous oxide, *Laryngoscope* 107(3):357, 1997.
40. Berthold M: Safety alert: nitrous oxide—screen for recent ophthalmic surgery, *ADA News* 6:20, 2002.
41. Hart RH *et al*: Loss of vision caused by expansion on intraocular perfluoropropane gas during nitrous oxide anesthesia, *Am J Ophthalmology* 134(5):761, 2002.

Chapter 10

Patient Assessment

To best serve the patient, it is imperative that the healthcare provider obtain an initial medical history from the patient. This information is acquired through a formal interview and updated at each visit. Undivided attention is necessary to assess the patient's physiological and psychological status so that the best pain and anxiety management option may be selected. The ASA Task Force[1] agrees that obtaining a preprocedure evaluation increases the likelihood of success during sedation and decreases the chance for adverse outcomes. Even friends and relatives who practitioners think they know well must have this formal scrutiny. Hence the familiar axiom: *Never treat a stranger.*

I. OBTAINING PATIENT HISTORY INFORMATION

A. The patient often completes questions about health and personal information in the reception area, with no further inquiries made by a practitioner. It is assumed that this information is seen before patient treatment; however, this may not always be the case.

B. It is advantageous to obtain this information through direct interaction with patients. Information exchanged through a formal interview enables practitioners to further question responses and make an assessment of patient pain and anxiety. The person directly involved with the treatment of the patient should complete the interview.

C. Information specific to sedation that should be collected includes (1) abnormalities of the major organ systems; (2) previous adverse experience with sedation or analgesia; (3) drug allergies, current medications, and potential drug interactions; (4) time and nature of last oral intake; and (5) history of tobacco, alcohol, or substance use or abuse.[1]

D. It is highly recommended to include a question(s) about pain and anxiety on the health history form itself.[2] This question provides patients with a nonthreatening way to communicate anxious feelings that they may be hesitant to divulge verbally. Examples of such questions include "Is there anything about being here for treatment that bothers you?" "Have you had a negative experience in an office or clinic before?" or "Have you previously required special procedures or medication for nervousness before an appointment?"

   1. Scales indicating pain and/or anxiety levels can be included on the health history form as well.

   2. Some patients will feel comfortable about communicating their anxious feelings verbally. Others will not admit to uncomfortable feelings but may show outward signs such as sweating, shaking, and syncope. In any case, those initial minutes of dialogue are valuable for gathering information.

E. A professional can then use the health information obtained from the interview to make an assessment about the health risk to the patient before performing a medical or dental procedure.

II. ASSESSMENT OF PATIENT RISK

A. The American Society of Anesthesiologists (ASA) developed a method of classifying patients according to medical risk. The Physical Status Classification system was initiated in the early 1960s and is recognized around the world.[3] Its applicability and validity for almost every health discipline are the reasons for its continued use today. During assessment of the health and physical status of patients, this system helps determine whether a patient is an appropriate candidate for sedation (Box 10-1).

B. The ASA Physical Status Classification system.[4]

    1. ASA I—Patients with no systemic disease. These patients are able to tolerate mild physical exertion and psychologic stresses. They do not possess any organic, physiologic, biochemical, or psychiatric disturbances. These patients may be considered appropriate candidates for N_2O/O_2 sedation.

    2. ASA II—Patients with mild-to-moderate physiologic disturbance that is under good control. There is no significant compromise of normal activity; however, the patient's specific condition could possibly affect the safety of surgery and anesthesia. Depending on their particular situation, these patients are usually considered appropriate candidates for N_2O/O_2 sedation.

    3. ASA III—Patients with a major systemic disturbance that is difficult to control. There is significant compromise of normal activity for this patient. This situation creates a significant impact on surgery and anesthesia. Medical consultation is recommended for these patients. These patients present greater risk for treatment; however, N_2O/O_2 sedation may still be used following medical advice.

    4. ASA IV—Patients with severe and potentially life-threatening systemic disease that significantly limits their activity are not usually seen in an ambulatory health setting. Because of their unstable health problems, they are categorized as high risk for many situations; the potential for an acute emergency situation is great. Seek medical consultation and/or referral. N_2O/O_2 is usually not indicated except in emergency situations.

    5. ASA V—Moribund patients in whom immediate surgery is the last effort to save their lives. In some cases, N_2O/O_2 is recommended for pain and anxiety relief in these final stages.

    6. ASA VI—The patient in this classification is clinically dead but being maintained for organ donation.

    7. ASA E—Designation for a patient in any ASA classification requiring an emergency procedure.

Box 10-1   ASA PHYSICAL STATUS DEFINITION

Classification of Physical Status

ASA I—A normal healthy patient

ASA II—A patient with mild systemic disease

ASA III—A patient with severe systemic disease

ASA IV—A patient with severe systemic disease that is a constant threat to life

ASA V—A moribund patient who is not expected to survive without an operation

ASA VI—A declared brain-dead patient whose organs are being removed for donor purposes

E—Patient requires emergency procedure

From the American Society of Anesthesiologists: *Manual for Anesthesia Department Organization and Management*, Park Ridge, IL, 2003, American Society of Anesthesiologists. Reprinted with permission of the American Society of Anesthesiologists, Park Ridge, Illinois.

III. PREPROCEDURAL PATIENT EVALUATION

A. **Vital signs**
   1. Evaluating preoperative, intraoperative, and postoperative vital signs is considered the standard of care by the ASA, ADSA, and several other health societies and organizations.[5] Vital sign values should be recorded in the patient's chart each time they are measured. It is appropriate to obtain baseline values at the initial visit and then periodically thereafter.
   2. Depending on the discipline, specialties with established guidelines for delivering anesthesia and sedation may recommend that vital signs be measured whenever N_2O/O_2 is used.[6-8] State governing bodies may also require that vital signs be measured.[9]
   3. There is a total of six vital signs: height, weight, body temperature, blood pressure, pulse, and respiration.
   4. Depending on the clinical setting and treatment being performed, some vital signs are measured more frequently than others. Blood pressure, pulse, and respiration are the most dynamic vital signs and should be recorded at each visit. Oxygen saturation level and a pain score have been advocated in some cases to be included with vital sign information.[10]
   5. Vital sign measurements recommended for minimal sedation are blood pressure, pulse, and respiration. These should be obtained preoperatively to provide a baseline reference before N_2O/O_2 administration. Postoperative vital signs serve as a measure of recovery from N_2O/O_2 sedation. These values are compared with those obtained preoperatively and are assessed for the degree of variation.
      a. Guidelines regarding hypertension and blood pressure indicators for adults have recently changed according to the National Heart, Lung, and Blood Institute. Normal blood pressure is classified as <120 mm Hg systolic and <80 mm Hg diastolic readings. Prehypertension is classified when systolic readings are within the range of 120–139 mm Hg or a diastolic reading within the range of 80–89 mm Hg. Stage 1 hypertension is when systolic readings are 140–159 mm Hg or a diastolic reading ranges from 90–99 mm Hg. Stage 2 hypertension is a systolic reading of >160 mm Hg or a diastolic value of >100 mm Hg. Dental procedures may be completed for those patients with Stage 1 hypertension; it is also suggested that nitrous oxide be used for anxious hypertensive patients.[11] It is not recommended to treat adults with extremely elevated blood pressure. Those patients should be immediately referred to a medical facility for evaluation (Table 10-1).
      b. The fourth report from the National High Blood Pressure Education Program Working Group on Children and Adolescents outlines the latest recommendations

Table 10-1. Blood Pressure Classification for Adults

Blood Pressure Classification	Systolic Blood Pressure (SBP mm Hg)	Diastolic Blood Pressure (DBP mm Hg)
Normal	< 120	< 80
Prehypertension	120–139	80–89
Stage 1 Hypertension	140–159	90–99
Stage 2 Hypertension	≥ 160	≥ 100

From the U.S. Department of Health and Human Services; National Institutes of Health: National Heart, Lung, and Blood Institute; National High Blood Pressure Education Program.

regarding hypertension in young persons.[12] This updated report includes revised blood pressure tables that can be used by healthcare providers as a reference. Blood pressure values for children and adolescents correlate with height and weight percentiles established for each gender. Normal blood pressure is defined as systolic and diastolic values that are less than the 90th percentile for gender, age, and height.[12] Hypertension for this population is defined as blood pressure values that are greater than or equal to the 95th percentile for gender, age, and height when taken on multiple occasions.[12] The growth charts and accompanying height and weight percentiles for both boys and girls are presented in this chapter for quick reference (see Figures 10-1 and 10-2 and Tables 10-2 and 10-3).

B. Auscultation of the heart and lungs and evaluation of the airway are recommended by the ASA Task Force before sedation.

   1. A precordial-pretracheal stethoscope is a simple, inexpensive, and excellent way to monitor respiration and heart sounds. The stethoscope head is weighted and can be secured in place with tape. The tubing connects to one or two earpieces. The pretracheal scope head is placed in the midline of the neck near the lower end of the trachea. At this location, sounds of air exchange can easily be heard. The scope can also be placed in the precordial region over the heart. At this location, both heart and lung sounds can be heard[13] (Figure 10-3).

   2. Preprocedure evaluation of the airway can uncover airway abnormalities that could increase the likelihood of airway obstruction.[1] The evaluation includes questioning the patient about previous problems with anesthesia or sedation, sleep problems, advanced rheumatoid arthritis, or chromosomal abnormalities. Physical evaluation includes the determination of size and limitations of the head, neck, and mouth, as well as variations in occlusion and teeth (Box 10-2).

   3. Remember, the operator must be prepared to manage the complications associated with the next (deeper) level of sedation beyond that which is intended.[1]

IV. PATIENT PREPARATION

A. It is not necessary to fast prior to N_2O/O_2 sedation. However, guidelines are provided as a reference (Box 10-3).

   1. It is not recommended that patients eat fatty, fried, or greasy foods just prior to N_2O/O_2 sedation. This is especially true with children.

   2. A light meal that includes carbohydrates is appropriate if eaten an hour or so prior to the procedure.

   3. Vomiting should not occur when N_2O/O_2 sedation is appropriately administered. It is necessary to be prepared for the adverse conditions that are associated with moderate sedation.

B. Before N_2O/O_2 sedation, the patient should be informed about the intent of the procedure and how it will be accomplished along with the risks, benefits, and alternatives to its use.[1,9]

   1. Informed consent should be obtained from competent patients and/or legal guardians of children or others each time N_2O/O_2 is administered.

   2. Although the law does not mandate written consent, it is advisable to have a specific form with the information followed by the patient's or guardian's signature and the date (Fig. 10-4). An example of a consent form appropriate for N_2O/O_2 administration can be found in Appendix D.

V. PATIENT MONITORING

During N_2O/O_2 sedation, it is necessary to continuously monitor the patient. This is to ensure a positive experience for the patient and to discover adverse reactions quickly. The ASA Task

(Text continues on page 109)

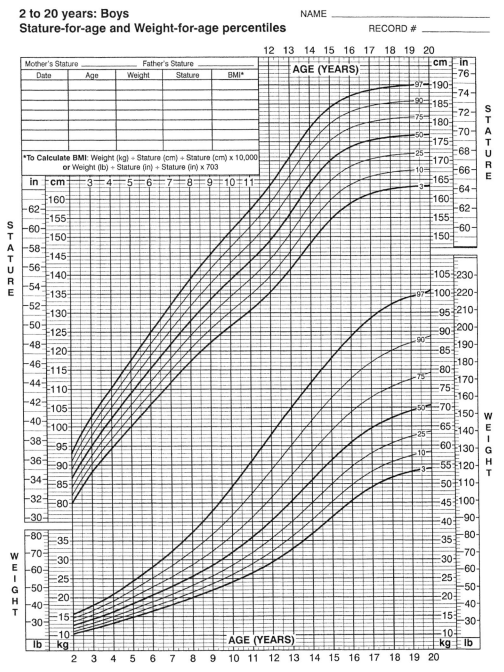

2 to 20 years: Boys
Stature-for-age and Weight-for-age percentiles

NAME _____

RECORD # _____

Figure 10-1 Growth chart for boys. BMI, body mass index. (*Developed by the National Center for Health Statistics in collaboration with the National Center for Chronic Disease Prevention and Health Promotion (2000).* http://www.cdc.gov/growthcharts).

2 to 20 years: Girls
Stature-for-age and Weight-for-age percentiles

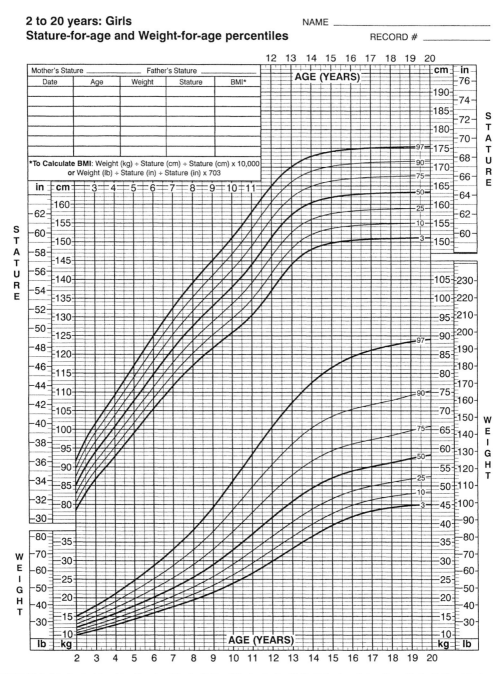

Figure 10-2 Growth chart for girls. *(Developed by the National Center for Health Statistics in collaboration with the National Center for Chronic Disease Prevention and Health Promotion (2000).* http://www.cdc.gov/growthcharts*).*

Table 10-2. Blood Pressure Levels for Boys by Age and Height Percentile*

Age (Years)	BP Percentile	Systolic BP (mm Hg) Percentile of Height							Diastolic BP (mm Hg) Percentile of Height						
		5th	10th	25th	50th	75th	90th	95th	5th	10th	25th	50th	75th	90th	95th
1	50th	80	81	83	85	87	88	89	34	35	36	37	38	39	39
	90th	94	95	97	99	100	102	103	49	50	51	52	53	53	54
	95th	98	99	101	103	104	106	106	54	54	55	56	57	58	58
	99th	105	106	108	110	112	113	114	61	62	63	64	65	66	66
2	50th	84	85	87	88	90	92	92	39	40	41	42	43	44	44
	90th	97	99	100	102	104	105	106	54	55	56	57	58	58	59
	95th	101	102	104	106	108	109	110	59	59	60	61	62	63	63
	99th	109	110	111	113	115	117	117	66	67	68	69	70	71	71
3	50th	86	87	89	91	93	94	95	44	44	45	46	47	48	48
	90th	100	101	103	105	107	108	109	59	59	60	61	62	63	63
	95th	104	105	107	109	110	112	113	63	63	64	65	66	67	67
	99th	111	112	114	116	118	119	120	71	71	72	73	74	75	75
4	50th	88	89	91	93	95	96	97	47	48	49	50	51	51	52
	90th	102	103	105	107	109	110	111	62	63	64	65	66	66	67
	95th	106	107	109	111	112	114	115	66	67	68	69	70	71	71
	99th	113	114	116	118	120	121	122	74	75	76	77	78	78	79
5	50th	90	91	93	95	96	98	98	50	51	52	53	54	55	55
	90th	104	105	106	108	110	111	112	65	66	67	68	69	69	70
	95th	108	109	110	112	114	115	116	69	70	71	72	73	74	74
	99th	115	116	118	120	121	123	123	77	78	79	80	81	81	82
6	50th	91	92	94	96	98	99	100	53	53	54	55	56	57	57
	90th	105	106	108	110	111	113	113	68	68	69	70	71	72	72
	95th	109	110	112	114	115	117	117	72	72	73	74	75	76	76
	99th	116	117	119	121	123	124	125	80	80	81	82	83	84	84

(Continued)

Table 10-2. Blood Pressure Levels for Boys by Age and Height Percentile*—cont'd

Age (Years)	BP Percentile	Systolic BP (mm Hg) Percentile of Height							Diastolic BP (mm Hg) Percentile of Height						
		5th	10th	25th	50th	75th	90th	95th	5th	10th	25th	50th	75th	90th	95th
7	50th	92	94	95	97	99	100	101	55	55	56	57	58	59	59
	90th	106	107	109	111	113	114	115	70	70	71	72	73	74	74
	95th	110	111	113	115	117	118	119	74	74	75	76	77	78	78
	99th	117	118	120	122	124	125	126	82	82	83	84	85	86	86
8	50th	94	95	97	99	100	102	102	56	57	58	59	60	60	61
	90th	107	109	110	112	114	115	116	71	72	72	73	74	75	76
	95th	111	112	114	116	118	119	120	75	76	77	78	79	79	80
	99th	119	120	122	123	125	127	127	83	84	85	86	87	87	88
9	50th	95	96	98	100	102	103	104	57	58	59	60	61	61	62
	90th	109	110	112	114	115	117	118	72	73	74	75	76	76	77
	95th	113	114	116	118	119	121	121	76	77	78	79	80	81	81
	99th	120	121	123	125	127	128	129	84	85	86	87	88	88	89
10	50th	97	98	100	102	103	105	106	58	59	60	61	61	62	63
	90th	111	112	114	115	117	119	119	73	73	74	75	76	77	78
	95th	115	116	117	119	121	122	123	77	78	79	80	81	81	82
	99th	122	123	125	127	128	130	130	85	86	86	88	88	89	90
11	50th	99	100	102	104	105	107	107	59	59	60	61	62	63	63
	90th	113	114	115	117	119	120	121	74	74	75	76	77	78	78
	95th	117	118	119	121	123	124	125	78	78	79	80	81	82	82
	99th	124	125	127	129	130	132	132	86	86	87	88	89	90	90
12	50th	101	102	104	106	108	109	110	59	60	61	62	63	63	64
	90th	115	116	118	120	121	123	123	74	75	75	76	77	78	79
	95th	119	120	122	123	125	127	127	78	79	80	81	82	82	83
	99th	126	127	129	131	133	134	135	86	87	88	89	90	90	91
13	50th	104	105	106	108	110	111	112	60	60	61	62	63	64	64
	90th	117	118	120	122	124	125	126	75	75	76	77	78	79	79
	95th	121	122	124	126	128	129	130	79	79	80	81	82	83	83
	99th	128	130	131	133	135	136	137	87	87	88	89	90	91	91

Age (Year)	BP Percentile*	SBP (mmHg) Percentile of Height							DBP (mmHg) Percentile of Height						
		5th	10th	25th	50th	75th	90th	95th	5th	10th	25th	50th	75th	90th	95th
14	50th	106	107	109	111	113	114	115	60	61	62	63	64	65	65
	90th	120	121	123	125	126	128	128	75	76	77	78	79	79	80
	95th	124	125	127	128	130	132	132	80	80	81	82	83	84	84
	99th	131	132	134	136	138	139	140	87	88	89	89	91	92	92
15	50th	109	110	112	113	115	117	117	61	62	63	64	65	66	66
	90th	122	124	125	128	129	130	131	76	77	78	79	80	80	81
	95th	126	127	129	131	133	134	135	81	81	82	83	84	85	85
	99th	134	135	136	138	140	142	142	88	89	90	91	92	93	93
16	50th	111	112	114	116	118	119	120	63	63	64	65	66	67	67
	90th	125	126	128	130	131	133	134	78	78	79	80	81	82	82
	95th	129	130	132	134	135	137	137	82	83	83	84	85	86	87
	99th	136	137	139	141	143	144	145	90	90	91	92	93	94	94
17	50th	114	115	116	118	120	121	122	65	66	66	67	68	69	70
	90th	127	128	130	132	134	135	136	80	80	81	82	83	84	84
	95th	131	132	134	136	138	139	140	84	85	86	87	88	88	89
	99th	139	140	141	143	145	146	147	92	93	93	94	95	96	97

The Fourth Report on the Diagnosis, Evaluation, and Treatment of High Blood Pressure in Children and Adolescents, *Pediatrics* 114(2 Suppl 4th Report):555–76, 2004.

BP, Blood pressure.

*The 90th percentile is 1.28 SD, the 95th percentile is 1.645 SD, and the 99th percentile is 2.326 SD over the mean. For research purposes, the standard deviations in Appendix B allow one to compute BP Z-scores and percentiles for boys with height percentiles given in Table 10-3 (i.e., the 5th, 10th, 25th, 50th, 75th, 90th and 95th percentiles). These height percentiles must be converted to height Z-scores given by (5%= -1.645; 10%= -1.28' 25%= -0.68; 50%= 0; 75%= 0.68; 90%= 1.28; 95%= 1.645) and then computed according to the methodology in steps 2–4 described in Appendix B. For children with height percentiles other than these, follow steps 1–4 described in Appendix B.

Table 10-3. Blood Pressure Levels for Girls by Age and Height Percentile*

Age (Years)	BP Percentile	Systolic BP (mm Hg) Percentile of Height							Diastolic BP (mm Hg) Percentile of Height						
		5th	10th	25th	50th	75th	90th	95th	5th	10th	25th	50th	75th	90th	95th
1	50th	83	84	85	86	88	89	90	38	39	39	40	41	41	42
	90th	97	97	98	100	101	102	103	52	53	53	54	55	55	56
	95th	100	101	102	104	105	106	107	56	57	57	58	59	59	60
	99th	108	108	109	111	112	113	114	64	64	65	65	66	67	67
2	50th	85	85	87	88	89	91	91	43	44	44	46	46	46	47
	90th	98	99	100	101	103	104	105	57	58	58	59	60	61	61
	95th	102	103	104	105	107	108	109	61	62	62	63	64	65	65
	99th	109	110	111	112	114	115	116	69	69	70	70	71	72	72
3	50th	86	87	88	89	91	92	93	47	48	48	49	50	50	51
	90th	100	100	102	103	104	106	106	61	62	62	63	64	64	65
	95th	104	104	105	107	108	109	110	65	66	66	67	68	68	69
	99th	111	111	113	114	115	116	117	73	73	74	74	75	76	76
4	50th	88	88	90	91	92	94	94	50	50	51	52	52	53	54
	90th	101	102	103	104	106	107	108	64	64	65	66	67	67	68
	95th	105	106	107	108	110	111	112	68	68	69	70	71	71	72
	99th	112	113	114	115	117	118	119	76	76	76	77	78	79	79
5	50th	89	90	91	93	94	95	96	52	53	53	54	55	55	56
	90th	103	103	105	106	107	109	109	66	67	67	68	69	69	70
	95th	107	107	108	110	111	112	113	70	71	71	72	73	73	74
	99th	114	114	116	117	118	120	120	78	78	79	79	80	81	81
6	50th	91	92	93	94	96	97	98	54	54	55	56	56	57	58
	90th	104	105	106	108	109	110	111	68	68	69	70	70	71	72
	95th	108	109	110	111	113	114	115	72	72	73	74	74	75	76
	99th	115	116	117	119	120	121	122	80	80	80	81	82	83	83

Age	BP Percentile														
7	50th	59	58	58	57	56	56	55	99	99	97	96	95	93	93
	90th	73	72	72	71	70	70	69	113	112	111	109	108	107	106
	95th	77	73	76	75	74	74	73	116	116	115	113	112	111	110
	99th	84	84	83	82	82	81	81	124	123	122	120	119	118	117
8	50th	60	60	59	58	57	57	57	101	100	99	98	96	95	95
	90th	74	74	73	72	71	71	71	114	114	113	111	110	709	108
	95th	78	78	77	76	75	75	75	118	118	116	115	114	112	112
	99th	86	85	84	83	83	82	82	125	125	123	122	121	120	119
9	50th	61	61	60	59	58	58	58	103	102	101	100	98	97	96
	90th	75	75	70	73	72	72	72	116	116	114	113	112	110	110
	95th	79	79	78	77	76	76	76	120	119	118	117	115	114	114
	99th	87	86	85	84	84	83	83	127	127	125	124	123	121	121
10	50th	62	62	61	60	59	59	59	105	104	103	102	100	99	98
	90th	76	76	75	74	73	73	73	118	118	116	115	114	112	112
	95th	80	80	79	78	77	77	77	122	121	120	119	117	116	116
	99th	87	87	86	86	84	84	84	129	129	127	126	125	123	123
11	50th	63	63	62	61	60	60	60	107	106	105	103	102	101	100
	90th	77	77	76	75	74	74	74	120	119	118	117	116	114	114
	95th	81	81	80	79	78	78	78	124	123	122	121	119	118	118
	99th	89	88	87	87	86	85	85	131	130	129	128	126	125	125
12	50th	64	67	63	62	61	61	61	109	108	107	105	104	103	102
	90th	78	78	77	76	75	75	75	122	121	120	119	117	116	116
	95th	82	82	81	81	79	79	79	126	125	124	123	121	120	119
	99th	90	89	88	89	87	86	86	133	132	131	130	128	127	127
13	50th	65	65	64	63	62	62	62	110	110	109	107	106	105	104
	90th	79	79	78	77	76	76	76	124	123	122	121	119	118	117
	95th	83	83	82	81	80	80	80	128	127	126	124	123	122	121
	99th	91	90	89	89	88	87	87	135	134	133	132	130	129	128
14	50th	66	66	65	64	63	63	63	112	111	110	109	107	106	106
	90th	80	80	79	78	77	77	77	125	125	124	122	121	120	119
	95th	84	84	83	82	81	81	81	129	129	127	126	125	123	123
	99th	92	91	90	90	89	88	88	136	136	135	133	132	131	130

(Continued)

Table 10-3. Blood Pressure Levels for Girls by Age and Height Percentile*—cont'd

Age (Years)	BP Percentile	Systolic BP (mm Hg) Percentile of Height							Diastolic BP (mm Hg) Percentile of Height						
		5th	10th	25th	50th	75th	90th	95th	5th	10th	25th	50th	75th	90th	95th
15	50th	107	108	109	110	111	113	113	64	64	64	65	66	67	67
	90th	120	121	122	123	125	126	127	78	78	78	79	80	81	81
	95th	124	125	126	127	129	130	131	82	82	82	83	84	85	85
	99th	131	132	133	134	136	137	138	89	89	90	91	91	92	93
16	50th	108	108	110	111	112	114	114	64	64	65	66	66	67	68
	90th	121	122	123	124	126	127	128	78	78	79	80	81	81	82
	95th	125	126	127	128	130	131	132	82	82	83	84	85	85	86
	99th	132	133	134	135	137	138	139	90	90	90	91	92	93	93
17	50th	108	109	110	111	113	114	115	64	65	65	66	67	67	68
	90th	122	122	123	125	126	127	128	78	79	79	80	81	81	82
	95th	125	126	127	128	130	131	132	82	83	83	84	85	85	86
	99th	133	133	134	136	137	138	139	90	90	91	91	92	93	93

The Fourth Report on the Diagnosis, Evaluation, and Treatment of High Blood Pressure in Children and Adolescents, *Pediatrics* 114(2 Suppl 4th Report):555–76, 2004.

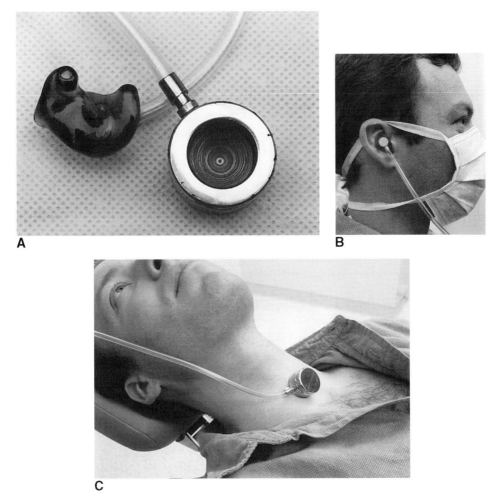

Figure 10-3 A, Pretracheal stethoscope and earpiece. **B,** Pretracheal earpiece placement. **C,** Pretracheal stethoscope placement. (*From Malamed SF:* Sedation: A Guide to Patient Management, *ed 4, St. Louis, 2003, Mosby.*)

Force recommends that monitoring the patient include evaluating level of consciousness, pulmonary ventilation, oxygenation, and hemodynamics.

A. Levels of consciousness can be monitored by the patient's response to verbal stimulation. Monitoring level of consciousness reduces risks associated with moderate sedation.

B. Monitoring ventilatory function can be accomplished by observation or auscultation. This reduces the risk of adverse outcomes associated with moderate sedation. A great advantage of N_2O/O_2 delivery is the reservoir bag. This serves as a supplemental supply of O_2 for the patient but also is a valid method of monitoring a patient's respiration. The bag mimics respiratory excursions, allowing the practitioner to monitor the frequency and depth of respirations with a reliable visual source.

C. Pulse oximetry detects oxygen desaturation and can uncover early hypoxemia. Early detection of hypoxemia through the use of a pulse oximeter decreases the likelihood of severe adverse reactions. Cyanosis is a late sign of respiratory distress.

Box 10-2 **AIRWAY ASSESSMENT PROCEDURES FOR SEDATION AND ANALGESIA**

Positive-pressure ventilation, with or without tracheal intubation, may be necessary if respiratory compromise develops during sedation-analgesia. This may be difficult in patients with atypical airway anatomy. In addition, some airway abnormalities may increase the likelihood of airway obstruction during spontaneous ventilation. Some factors that may be associated with difficulty in airway management are the following:

History
Previous problems with anesthesia or sedation
Stridor, snoring, or sleep apnea
Advanced rheumatoid arthritis
Chromosomal abnormality (e.g., trisomy 21)

Physical examination

Habitus
Significant obesity (especially involving the neck and facial structures)

Head and neck
Short neck, limited neck extension, decreased hyoid-mental distance (<3 cm in an adult), neck mass, cervical spine disease or trauma, tracheal deviation, dysmorphic facial features (e.g., Pierre-Robin syndrome)

Mouth
Small opening (<3 cm in an adult), edentulous, protruding incisors, loose or capped teeth, dental appliances, high arched palate, macroglossia, tonsillar hypertrophy, nonvisible uvula

Jaw
Micrognathia, retrognathia, trismus, significant malocclusion

Modified from ASA Task Force: Practice guidelines for sedation and analgesia by non-anesthesiologists, *Anesthesiology* 96(4):1004, 2005–2006. Reprinted with permission of the American Society of Anesthesiologists, Park Ridge, Illinois.

Box 10-3 **PREPROCEDURE FASTING GUIDELINES**

Ingested Material	Minimum Fasting Period
Clear liquid	2 hours
Nonhuman milk	6 hours
Light meals	6 hours

These recommendations apply to healthy patients who are undergoing elective procedures. They are not intended for women in labor. Following the guidelines does not guarantee complete gastric emptying has occurred.

The fasting periods apply to all ages.

Examples of clear liquids include water, fruit juices without pulp, carbonated beverages, clear tea, and black coffee.

Because nonhuman milk is similar to solids in gastric emptying time, the amount ingested must be considered when determining an appropriate fasting period.

A light meal typically consists of toast and clear liquids. Meals that include fried or fatty foods or meat may prolong gastric emptying time. Both the amount and type of food ingested must be considered when determining an appropriate fasting period.

Modified from ASA Task Force: Practice guidelines for sedation and analgesia by non-anesthesiologists, *Anesthesiology* 96(4):1004, 2005–2006. Reprinted with permission of the American Society of Anesthesiologists, Park Ridge, Illinois.

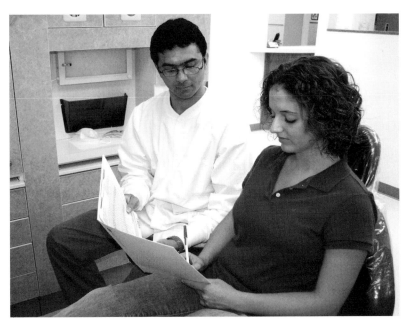

Figure 10-4 Obtain informed consent from the patient prior to sedation.

VI. EMERGENCY PREPAREDNESS

A. Personnel preparation

1. Persons who are involved in the administration and monitoring of N_2O/O_2 sedation should understand the pharmacokinetics and pharmacodynamics of the drug and be able to recognize complications.

2. Personnel who use N_2O/O_2 sedation and/or local anesthesia should be certified in basic life support that includes CPR and management of airway obstruction for adults, children, and infants.[9]

B. Emergency equipment

1. Appropriate emergency equipment should be readily available wherever patients are treated. The ASA Task Force recommends that an automated external defibrillator (AED) should be available when moderate sedation is intended.[1]

2. Additional equipment that is recommended includes antagonist medications, a positive-pressure ventilation system, adequate suction to clear an airway, advanced airway equipment, and resuscitation medications.[1,9]

3. These items are standard for those who administer sedation.

REFERENCES

1. ASA Task Force: Practice guidelines for sedation and analgesia by non-anesthesiologists, *Anesthesiology* 96 (4):1004, 2002.
2. Wolfe S: The practical approach to painless dentistry, *Dentistry Today* 11:30, 1992.
3. American Society of Anesthesiologists: New classification of physical status, *Anesthesiology* 24:111, 1963.
4. Sweitzer B: *Handbook of Preoperative Assessment and Treatment*, Philadelphia, 2000, Lippincott Williams & Wilkins.

5. American Academy of Pediatric Dentistry: Standards for basic intraoperative monitoring, *ASA Newsletter* 50:13, 1986.

6. American Association of Oral and Maxillofacial Surgeons, Committee on Anesthesia: *Office Anesthesia Evaluation Manual,* ed 4, Rosemont, Ill, 1991, The Association.

7. American Academy of Pediatric Dentistry: Guidelines for the elective use of conscious sedation, deep sedation, and general anesthesia in pediatric patients, *Pediatrics* 76:317, 1985.

8. American Academy of Periodontology: Subcommittee on Anxiety and Pain Control of the Pharmacotherapeutics Committee: *Guidelines for the Use of Conscious Sedation in Periodontics,* Chicago, 1990, The Association.

9. American Dental Association, Council on Dental Education and Licensure: *Guidelines for the Use of Conscious Sedation, Deep Sedation, and General Anesthesia for Dentists,* Chicago, 2002, American Dental Association.

10. Theil D: *Personal communication,* October 2002.

11. Herman WW *et al*: New national guidelines on hypertension: a summary for dentistry, *JADA* 135:576, 2004.

12. National High Blood Pressure Education Program Working Group on Children and Adolescents: *The Fourth Report on the Diagnosis, Evaluation, and Treatment of High Blood Pressure in Children and Adolescents,* 2006, U.S. Department of Health and Human Services.

13. Malamed SF: *Sedation: A Guide to Patient Management,* ed 4, St. Louis, 2003, Mosby, p 65.

Titration of N_2O/O_2 Gases

Titration is a method of administering a drug in incremental amounts until a desired endpoint is reached (Box 11-1). For N_2O/O_2 sedation, N_2O is given in incremental doses until a patient has reached a comfortable, relaxed state of sedation. The ability to titrate N_2O is a significant advantage because it allows the specific amount of drug that is required by that patient to be delivered. If titration is done properly, the patient does not receive any more of the drug than is necessary. Occasionally, patients have had negative experiences with N_2O/O_2 sedation. In such cases, the operator most likely did not titrate properly; instead, the patient may have received an inappropriate amount of drug. The concept of titration is the single most important skill to be learned by the operator to be a competent, safe administrator of any drug by any route, including N_2O (Figure 11-1). The 2006 joint guidelines of the AAP and AAPD state that "the concept of titration of drug to effect is critical" and specifies that practitioners must know the full effect of a drug dosage before adding another.[1] *The titration technique is regarded as the current standard of care when administering N_2O/O_2 for sedation.*

The use of a rapid induction technique for N_2O/O_2 administration has been advocated by some clinicians for years. This technique involves administering a large quantity of N_2O (up to 50%) initially to patients, particularly children. Advocates of this technique maintain it is necessary to quickly calm an intensely fearful or uncooperative child. This technique in skilled hands can produce favorable results. The rapid induction technique is not recommended for adults. Pinkham[2] describes in the text *Pediatric Dentistry: Infancy through Adolescence* that the use of high concentrations with a rapid administration technique produces many negative effects.

The use of a 50% N_2O and 50% O_2 product may be a common practice for some. Seasoned clinicians and researchers Gillman and Lichtigfeld[3] advocate the use of the titration technique and advise others that they may have improved success rates when they use this technique instead of a 50% premixed concentration. It is therefore recommended that the rapid induction of high concentrations of N_2O not be used with adults and only with children under specific conditions and by a trained pediatric clinician.

I. SIGNIFICANCE

A. It is extremely desirable to provide only the amount of a drug necessary for the procedure being performed. This allows for the elimination of the drug from the system, but, more importantly, it creates a positive experience for the patient. With careful titration, vigilant monitoring of the patient, and updated equipment, negative experiences with N_2O/O_2 sedation should be rare.

> **Box 11-1** **TITRATION IS...**
>
> a method of drug administration in a substance is given in incremental doses until a specific desired clinical end-point is reached.

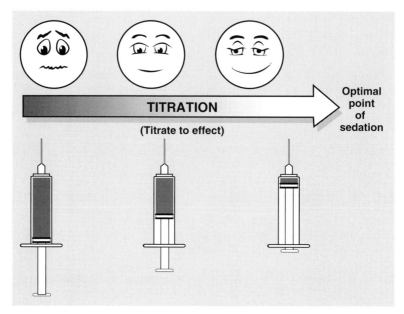

Figure 11-1 Titration is the incremental dosing of a drug. Incremental doses of a drug are administered to achieve an optimal point of sedation.

B. Titration is very important when administering any drug. It minimizes the chances of a severe, possibly life-threatening reaction should the patient be allergic to the drug. Since the discovery of N_2O, no allergic reaction to the drug has ever been reported.

C. Titration allows for biologic variability. It is essential to treat each patient as an individual, taking into account the concept of individual biovariability. This concept is based on the premise that no two individuals react the same way in response to a drug or treatment modality. What works for one will not necessarily work for another, nor will an individual respond in the same way on different days.

1. As each drug is initially tested, researchers commonly find a small percentage of hyporesponders and hyperresponders. Certain people will have no effect from an optimal dose of the drug, whereas some will incur dramatic effects. A drug is more efficacious when the desired outcome occurs in most of the population without unwanted side effects. Figure 11-2 depicts the range of individual biovariability.

2. Individual biovariability holds true for nonpharmacologic methods as well. It is wise to keep an open, informed mind when experimenting with pain and anxiety management options.

3. No two humans are alike, and the same individual may give a different response on any given day. For example, habitually dispensing 10 mg diazepam (Valium), 50 mg

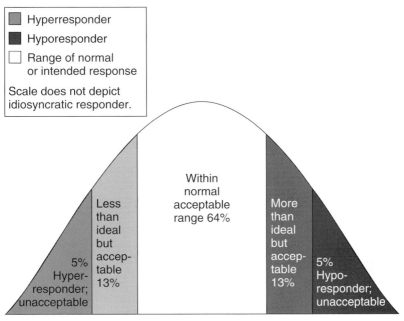

Figure 11-2 Range of individual biovariability.

meperidine (Demerol), or the use of 40% N_2O as a "usual" dose must be avoided, because patient response will not be standardized.

D. Sometimes idiosyncratic (unpredictable) reactions may be encountered that are untoward and inexplicable (e.g., excitement after receiving a sedative drug). Titrating the drug uncovers such responses and minimizes unexpected reactions (Box 11-2).

E. Titration can be applied to other drugs as well. For example, staggering local anesthetic injections over time allow for biotransformation tailored to the procedure and the patient's physiology. Titrating the dose of a drug is the considerate way to treat a patient individually. Titrating a drug to the appropriate level of sedation is a valuable learned skill.

II. ADJUSTING LEVELS APPROPRIATELY

A. A great advantage of N_2O is the ability to adjust levels of sedation. Because of this important pharmacologic property, the onset of clinical effects is rapid. Signs and symptoms of sedation may be missed if the patient is not closely monitored.

Box 11-2 ADVANTAGES OF N_2O TITRATION

- Only the amount of drug required by the patient is given.
- Allows for individual biovariability.
- Uncovers idiosyncratic reactions early.
- Minimizes negative experiences with oversedation.

B. Titration also allows for prolonged procedures to be accomplished effectively.

1. For example, when a potentially painful phase of treatment approaches, the N_2O gas may be increased. Conversely, as the intensity of the treatment subsides, the N_2O gas can be decreased.

2. As the procedure nears completion, amounts of N_2O being delivered should be discontinued and replaced with 100% O_2. Because a minimum of 5 minutes of post-oxygenation is required, it is appropriate to terminate the flow of N_2O and deliver 100% O_2 before completion of the procedure to expedite the recovery period.

C. Remember that because of individual biovariability, patients will require different levels of N_2O on different days and for different procedures.

1. The percentage of N_2O noted in a patient's chart from the last visit is not relevant for the current appointment.

2. A common mistake made with N_2O/O_2 sedation is to automatically deliver a preset percentage of N_2O to a patient.

3. Negative patient experiences from N_2O/O_2 sedation are most likely because the patient was oversedated as a result of operator error. Far too often patients blame any negative experience on the drug itself.

D. Regarding titration within the technique of N_2O/O_2 sedation, it is critical that once signs and symptoms of sedation begin to appear, it is critical that the patients' responses are closely monitored and time is given for doses to reach their peak effect. More information on the technique of N_2O/O_2 sedation is given in Chapter 13.

REFERENCES

1. AAP/AAPD Clinical Report: Guidelines for monitoring and management of pediatric patients during and after sedation for diagnostic and therapeutic procedures: an update, *Pediatrics* 118(6):2587, December 2006.
2. Pinkham JR, Casamassimo PS, McTigue DJ, Fields HW, Nowak A: *Pediatric Dentistry: Infancy through Adolescence*, ed 4, St. Louis, 2005, WB Saunders.
3. Gillman MA, Lichtigfeld FJ: Analgesic nitrous oxide: an opioid treatment for migraine, *Am J Emerg Med* 18 (4):501, 2000.

Signs and Symptoms of N_2O/O_2 Sedation

I ndividual biovariability accounts for different reactions to various amounts of N_2O. Some individuals experience several symptoms; others only a few. Symptoms are intense for some and insignificant for others. In some instances, signs are obvious; other times, signs are subtle. It is extremely important that the clinician knows what signs and symptoms to look for when administering and monitoring N_2O/O_2 sedation. Keeping a constant vigil is imperative, because pleasant sensations may quickly become unpleasant. Knowledge of the appropriate technique and associated physical, physiologic, and psychological changes increases the practitioner's confidence with the procedure and minimizes negative patient experiences. **The ultimate goal is to increase patient comfort through relaxation.**

I. APPROPRIATE MINIMAL SEDATION

A. A desirable level of sedation for both patient and operator using N_2O/O_2 sedation can be achieved by the use of the titration-time technique plus careful monitoring of the patient's signs and symptoms. Certain physical, physiologic, and psychological effects may manifest in individuals when N_2O and O_2 are administered (Box 12-1).

B. It is imperative that the operator recognize when the desired effects are reached, because it is then that an appropriate level of sedation is accomplished, and administration of additional drug is not necessary. The operator must watch closely for the following:

1. Psychological signs
   a. The patient is relaxed and comfortable (Figure 12-1).
   b. If asked, the patient acknowledges a reduced sense of fear and anxiety.
   c. The patient's mood may be categorized as happy, pleasant, satisfied, or even ambivalent (Figure 12-2).

2. Body movement
   a. Relaxation may be expressed overtly or inadvertently through physical movements. Signs of relaxation may include shoulders dropping, legs uncrossing, and arms laying looser on arm rests.
   b. Patients usually take deeper respirations when they are relaxed. A deep sigh or large inhalation may signal the patient is relaxing.

3. Eyes
   a. The activity of the patient's eyes is a good indicator of the level of sedation. With experience, the operator will often be able to make accurate judgments about the level of sedation by looking at the patient's eyes.
   b. Initially, during preparatory steps, patients' eyes will be active. Patients will be alert, and their eyes will follow the operator's actions and movements. This purposeful activity may lessen with sedation, as patients are no longer focused on the activities of others.

Box 12-1	SIGNS AND SYMPTOMS OF APPROPRIATE N_2O/O_2 SEDATION

Patient is comfortable and relaxed.
Patient acknowledges reduced fear and anxiety.
Patient is aware of surroundings.
Patient responds to directions and conversation.
Eyes become less active and glazed look appears.

Patient may experience:
   Tingling in extremities and/or near mouth
   Heaviness in legs and arms
   Body warmth
   Light feeling
   Vasodilation in face and neck
   Circumoral numbness

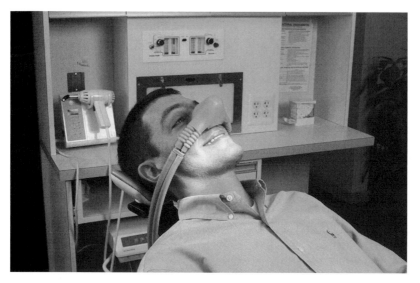

Figure 12-1 The patient is relaxed and comfortable.

    c. As sedation begins, the activity of the patient's eyes will begin to slow. Eye movement will be reduced, and blink rate will be slower (Figure 12-3). Although not recommended, patients may indicate their eyes are heavy and want to close them.

    d. As sedation continues, there will be a point, often, when the eyes may appear "glazed" or "glassy."

4. Facial expression

    a. Patients who are appropriately sedated are content. There is more of a "flat" expression rather than one that is "alert."

    b. There should not be signs of tension on the patient's face. The patient's forehead is a good place to look for tension and subsequent relaxation. When a patient is relaxed, muscles in the forehead and brow area should not be tight or strained.

    c. Patients will also smile easily. Smiles may come during questioning about how they are feeling or patients will smile without conversation. The smile correlates with a happy, joyful mood. Patients may also "giggle a little." They may say they "just can't help but smile" followed by a short, slight, laugh.

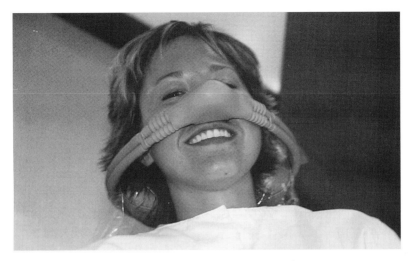

Figure 12-2 The patient is in a positive mood.

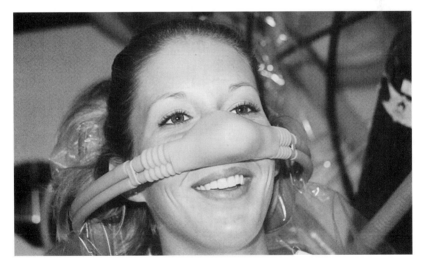

Figure 12-3 The patient's eye movement will be reduced.

5. Awareness
    a. When appropriately sedated, patients are fully conscious and aware of their surroundings. With relaxation, patients' surroundings are no longer threatening, and patients will have a sense of well-being.

    b. Patients will be able to respond rationally and coherently to the operator's inquiry or directions. They can maintain conversation. With N_2O/O_2 sedation, protective cough and gag reflexes remain intact. It is important to stress that patients refrain from talking to receive the drug's effects and minimize contamination of the environment.

    c. If a local anesthetic injection is given during the procedure, the operator can test the patient's level of sedation by asking, "Would this be a good time to give you the injection?" Patients will affirm the injection can be given when they are appropriately sedated and will be accepting of the procedure.

Anecdotally, the success of this questioning has proven to be quite reliable in clinical practice.

6. Other physiologic signs and symptoms

   a. Patients should not be given specific physical signs to expect such as tingling in the fingers, toes, cheeks, lips, tongue, head, or chest area. Some patients experience tingling sensations, but others may not. Therefore, the operator should not pose questions as to the presence of this symptom. Patients may think they are not being affected by the drug because they lack this symptom. Questions should be goal-oriented, focusing on how the patient is feeling rather than what the patient is feeling. It is important to indicate that a tingling sensation is a normal sensation with this sedation and not something that warrants concern. It is common for a patient to experience circumoral numbness.

   b. There may be noted heaviness in the patient's thighs and/or legs. Patients may associate this feeling to that when relaxing in an easy chair or just before going to sleep. Conversely, some patients experience a lighter feeling in their extremities. Again, these can be symptoms associated with sedation, and they should not warrant fear.

   c. Because of the drug's effect on the tympanic membrane, the patient's voice may resonate or carry a hypernasal tone. In addition, the patient may sense that the operator's voice is farther away and therefore harder to hear. Fabijan et al[1] challenge the idea that hearing acuity is changed with low levels of N_2O, but they indicate that the perception of the loudness of sounds is diminished.

   d. Patients may notice they feel warm. Their cheeks and/or neck may flush as vasodilation occurs. This degree of warmth should be one that is comfortable rather than uncomfortable.

II. OVERSEDATION

A. Discomfort in patients. As N_2O concentrations are increased, the signs and symptoms of comfort and relaxation may disappear. Some sensations may continue to be tolerable but become intense. Sometimes, changes in patient comfort occur rapidly, and a patient can suddenly become uncomfortable. In either case, the patient is no longer in a relaxed state. When a patient becomes uncomfortable in any way, it is important to decrease N_2O concentrations immediately. It is critical to regain patient comfort as soon as possible to avoid a significant negative experience.

B. Signs and symptoms of oversedation may not always be visually obvious. The operator should always be present whenever N_2O is being delivered to continuously monitor the patient. Patients should be told to signal or tell the operator if, at any point, they become uncomfortable. In addition, the operator should ask questions of patients periodically to assess comfort. The following are examples of the signs and symptoms of oversedation (Box 12-2).

1. Psychological signs

   a. The relaxed, comfortable state has disappeared.

      i. Patients may indicate that they just don't feel the same and that the effects such as tingling have intensified. This feeling may be annoying but not uncomfortable (Figure 12-4).

      ii. Or, the patient may indicate a sudden, very uncomfortable feeling in which symptoms are intolerable.

   b. In some cases, the patient may actually begin dreaming and/or hallucinating. Patients may attempt to respond to voices, people, visual effects, etc.

   c. Sexual fantasizing may occur with oversedation. The ramifications of this occurrence are discussed in Chapter 18.

Box 12-2	SIGNS AND SYMPTOMS OF OVERSEDATION

Detachment/disassociation from environment
Dreaming, hallucinating, or fantasizing
Out-of-body experiences
Floating and/or flying
Inability to move, communicate, or keep mouth open
Humming or vibrating sounds that progressively
  worsen

Patient may experience:
  Drowsiness
  Dizziness
  Diaphoresis
  Nausea
  Light-headedness
  Fixed eyes
  Uncomfortable body warmth

Patient may progress to:
  Sluggish, delayed responses
  Slurred words or no verbal sense
  Agitated or combative behavior
  Vomiting
  Unconsciousness

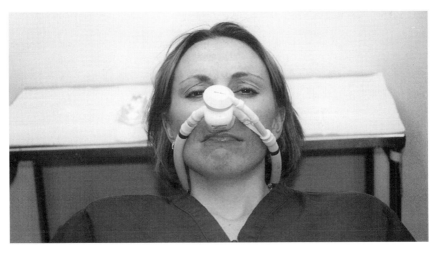

Figure 12-4 Oversedation; patient is irritated and uncomfortable.

2. Body movement
   a. Patients may show signs of being agitated or physically uncomfortable. They may become restless and fidgety.
   b. Patients can possibly become combative.
   c. Patients can also become very sluggish with their motions or unable to move their extremities.
3. Eyes
   a. The eyes of an oversedated patient can become fixed and nonresponsive.
   b. Heavily sedated patients often want to sleep and have difficulty keeping their eyes open.
   c. Occasionally, patients indicate their field of vision narrows. The area of their peripheral vision becomes black. Patients may comment that they feel like they are "blacking out."

4. Facial expression
    a. Fits of uncontrolled laughter are a sign of oversedation. When this occurs, the patient primarily mouth breathes, which changes the level of sedation.
    b. After the patient becomes calm and nose breathing resumes, a roller coaster sedation effect may occur and nausea can ensue.
5. Awareness
    a. Patients may no longer feel that they are in the same surroundings. A detachment or disassociation from the environment is possible.
    b. Often patients indicate lightweight, floating, or flying sensations. These may accompany the environmental detachment.
    c. Disassociation or out-of-body experiences can occur.
6. Other physiologic signs and symptoms
    a. Patients' perception of their hearing may change. The patient may perceive normal sounds as very intense. Humming noises or vibrations in their ears may simply be distracting or become bothersome.
    b. The pleasant warmth felt in earlier states might intensify and become uncomfortable. The patient may express various signs of being too warm or even hot. Wanting to loosen a collar or roll up sleeves may be indicators of perceived temperature increase.
    c. The patient may become very drowsy, which is not to be confused with being relaxed. The patient may actually want to sleep or appear to be in a dreamlike state.
    d. Words may be slurred or repeated; sentences may not be coherent. The patient may not be able to respond to verbal commands.
    e. Dizziness, light-headedness, and spinning sensations are common in oversedation. This may produce transient nausea for some patients.
    f. The tingling sensations felt in their extremities may now be felt throughout their body. This may feel similar to a shaking sensation.

C. Oversedation can produce physical and physiologic effects that are serious.
    1. Vomiting may occur with oversedation.
        a. Vomiting occurs more readily in children.
        b. Silent regurgitation is a type of action in which vomitus reaches the level of the epiglottis and can lead to aspiration into the lungs. This situation demands immediate advanced medical attention.
    2. The patient can actually become unconscious. Although this is difficult to do because of the pharmacokinetics of N_2O, all healthcare personnel must be able to respond to this type of emergency (see Chapter 8).
    3. These situations can easily be prevented with the titration technique with continuous monitoring.

D. When a patient has a pleasant experience when N_2O/O_2 sedation is used and the goal of analgesia and reduced anxiety is reached, success is achieved. However, oversedation typically produces a negative experience. Oversedation is likely when an inappropriate technique (i.e., fixed-dose, rapid induction) is applied or when equipment is used that only delivers a preset amount of drug. Patients who have had negative experiences with N_2O will, most often, not want to use the drug again. Conscientious, informed practitioners will not allow oversedation to destroy the capability of N_2O and O_2 to remain a viable option for pain and anxiety management.

REFERENCE

1. Fabijan DJ *et al*: The effect of nitrous oxide on hearing, *Anaesth Intensive Care* 28(3):270, 2000.

Technique for N₂O/O₂ Administration

T he basic principles of N_2O/O_2 administration have been developed from decades of experience. Adhering to these principles helps to ensure a positive experience for both the patient and the operator. Titrating the drug and careful observation of patient response are keys to successful administration. It is extremely important to know the fundamentals of the technique for administering N_2O/O_2. If these basic principles are followed, it will result in a positive experience for both the operator and the patient. If these basic principles are not followed, negative patient experiences can result. Concomitantly, operator frustration and lack of confidence occurred. It may take several positive experiences for a patient to become convinced that previous uncomfortable experiences were caused not by the N_2O but rather by its method of administration. **The technique is not difficult; titrating the drug while observing patient response is the key to success.**

I. FUNDAMENTAL PRINCIPLES FOR APPROPRIATE ADMINISTRATION

A. The operator should be enthusiastic and confident that the experience will be positive. This attitude will transfer to the patient.

B. Confidence is primarily preparation reflected in the individual who is informed and educated about N_2O pharmacokinetics. Be knowledgeable about what N_2O can and cannot accomplish.

C. Recognize that a patient in your care represents the best opportunity you have to express genuine care and concern. Patients are more likely to refer others to you after a good experience.

D. Informed consent must be obtained from each patient before each N_2O/O_2 administration.

E. The amount of N_2O required by a patient on any given day or time varies. Do not adopt the fixed-dose philosophy; the amount of N_2O required on the previous visit is not relevant for this appointment (see Chapter 11).

F. The procedure begins and ends with 100% pure O_2.

G. The patient should not be left alone. The effects of central nervous system depression may be quick and/or subtle; constant monitoring must be done by a professional trained in N_2O/O_2 sedation. Remember, you are responsible for the effects that occur at the intended level of sedation and the next (deeper) level.

H. Accurate documentation of all procedures must be maintained in the patient's file.

I. Because the final objective of the procedure is patient comfort, the patient should be placed in a comfortable position.

   1. To begin, depending on the discipline and the area of the body to be treated, the patient should be relaxed in a basic physiologic position.

2. The upper torso should be slightly reclined and the legs slightly elevated. This can be easily accomplished with an adjustable chair. If a bed is used, prop the patient with pillows.

J. Maintain open communication with the patient. Sedated patients may not be able to accurately state their feelings. Specific questions are necessary to assess the patient. For example, you may ask, "Are you uncomfortable?" or "On a scale of 1 to 10, what is your level of comfort?"

K. If N_2O/O_2 is to be given at a subsequent appointment, the patient should be advised to avoid eating a big meal that includes fatty, fried foods before that appointment.

II. GENERAL UNIT PREPARATION

A. The N_2O/O_2 sedation armamentarium should include all equipment necessary to provide safe sedation experiences for the patient and a safe environment for the operator and all other exposed personnel. Equipment should be evaluated for efficiency and integrity on a periodic basis.
1. This equipment should be current, accurate, and include all components for minimizing trace gas contamination (i.e., scavenging system).
2. A scavenging system will include an accurate flowmeter, scavenging masks, and a vacuum system able to eliminate gases at a rate of at least 45 L per minute.[2]

B. Ensure vacuum and ventilation exhaust are vented to the outside; make sure they are not near fresh-air intake vents.[2]

C. Assess the room and area ventilation.[2] The recirculation of room air, such as air conditioning, is not recommended to remove trace gas. A ventilation system with a fresh-air exchange system ensures that waste gases are not circulated elsewhere within the building.

D. Confirm the absence of leaks at pressure connections on the unit. Bubbles will appear at leaking locations when a soap and water solution is used. The hand-held unit available can quickly assess connections at the flowmeter for leaks (Figure 13-1).
1. Each time a cylinder is changed, checking the connections for leaks is also recommended. An inadequate seal will produce an audible hissing sound.
2. High-pressure lines should also be assessed periodically. The ADA expert panel recommends that this be done quarterly.[2]

E. Inspect the conducting tubing, reservoir bag, and their connections for leaks. Reservoir bags can tear if pulled off by the bag. Sterilizing tubing and bags will decrease their life. Make sure to have replacements on hand.

F. Connect the conducting tubing and reservoir bag to the unit if they are not already in place.

III. ACTIVATING N_2O/O_2 EQUIPMENT

A. Open both the O_2 and N_2O cylinders.
1. Turn the knob counterclockwise on the top of the large cylinders used in a central gas supply system. Open the stem valves on the top of smaller cylinders associated with a portable system (Figure 13-2). Pressure dials will show the contents of cylinders when the tanks are opened (Figure 13-3).
2. A central supply manifold should automatically switch the system to a full O_2 tank should one become depleted (Figure 13-4). If no additional O_2 is available for a central system, an alarm will sound or indicator light will flash on the system monitor. If there is no gas for the system, the lack of O_2 will automatically stop the flow of N_2O, and gas will cease flowing to the patient. The sedation machine becomes inoperable.

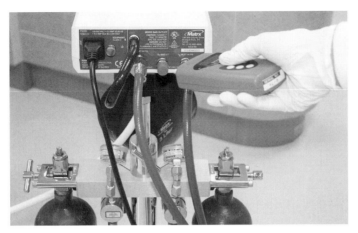

Figure 13-1 Checking connections on the flowmeter for leaks.

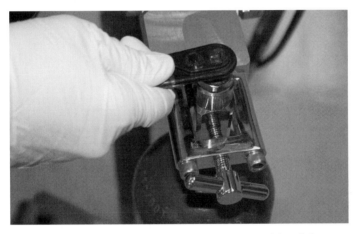

Figure 13-2 Open the O_2 tank by turning the valve on top of the cylinder.

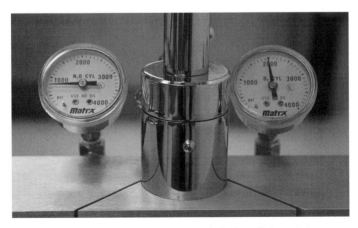

Figure 13-3 N_2O and O_2 pressure gauges indicating cylinder contents.

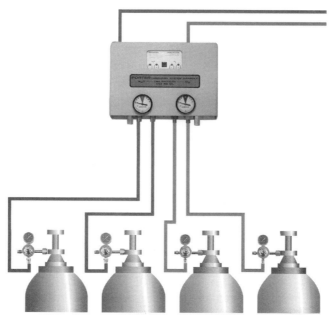

Figure 13-4 Pressure gauges on manifold. *(Courtesy of Porter Instrument Co.)*

3. The operator managing a portable system has to visually monitor the O_2 pressure gauge and manually replace cylinders when the oxygen supply is getting low. It is important to have a second cylinder readily available and opened before the oxygen is completely depleted to prevent loss of gas flow and interruption of patient sedation.
B. A bag barrier may be used to cover the unit; however, make sure the flowmeter can be easily read and knobs are easily accessible through the barrier (Figure 13-5).
C. Make sure the master switch on the flowmeter is in the "on" position.
D. Activate the main portion of the scavenging system by turning on the suction or evacuation system to the appropriate level.
1. This level may be automatically preset for some central supply systems. In this case, no further adjustments are necessary.
2. In some central supply systems, it is necessary to attach the end of the conduction tubing into the suction at the operatory.
3. For portable systems, it is necessary to place the tubing end into the high-speed suction (Figure 13-6).
4. If manual adjustment of the suction is necessary, create enough flow to prevent waste gas from entering the atmosphere. Manufacturing companies are currently marketing monitoring devices that indicate the optimal evacuation level of 45 L/min. Devices may be mounted close to the flowmeter; others may be found at the end of the conduction tubing before it is placed into the vacuum. The dependability of these devices can vary. An adequate level is achieved when the suction is audible (Figure 13-7).

IV. PATIENT PARTICIPATION

A. Review the patient's health history and obtain informed consent.
B. Measure the baseline vital signs of blood pressure (Figure 13-8, *A*), pulse (Figure 13-8, *B*), and respirations. Record these values on the sedation record or in the patient's chart.

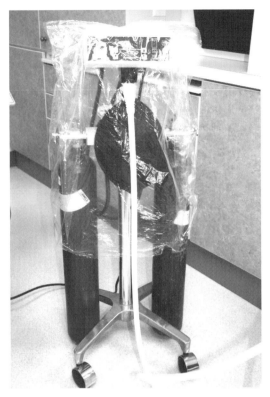

Figure 13-5 Bag barrier for disinfection.

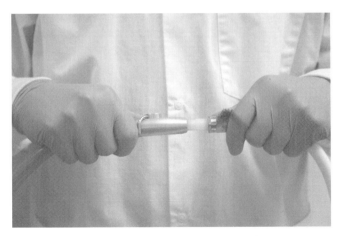

Figure 13-6 Engaging the delivery unit to the evacuation system.

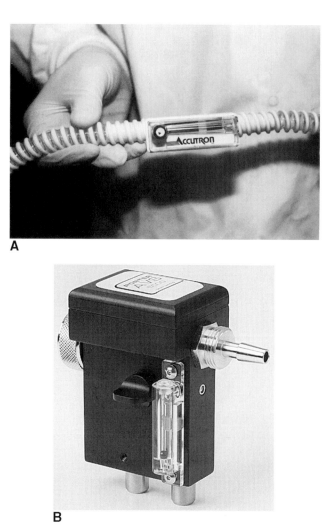

Figure 13-7 A and **B**, Devices used to monitor suction level. *(**A,** Courtesy of Accutron, Inc.; **B,** Courtesy of Porter Instrument Company.)*

C. Select the appropriate size and type of scavenging nasal hood for the patient. Find the size that fits the patients; the patient may select a scented or unscented variety. Attach breathing apparatus to conduction tubing.

D. Begin O_2 flow to the nasal hood or mask. The ball will float or the light will appear on the O_2 side of the flowmeter.

E. Estimate the total liters flow per minute (L/min) according to the size and physical and physiologic condition of the patient.

 1. For an average-size adult, begin with 6–7 L/min (Figure 13-9). It is best to err with more flow than needed initially to avoid a suffocating feeling. As the patient becomes relaxed, you may find that less flow is adequate.

 2. Begin with 4–5 L/min for most children.

 3. Set the machine to deliver 100% O_2 at the level of liters per minute that you have initially chosen. To ensure that there is flow, listen for the sound of O_2 moving into the breathing apparatus.

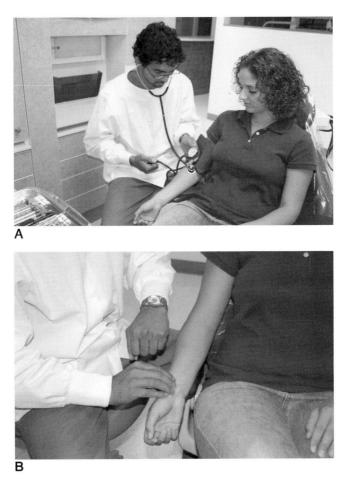

A

B

Figure 13-8 **A** and **B**, Obtain a blood pressure reading and pulse rate.

F. Push the O_2 flush button until the reservoir bag is partially inflated to approximately two-thirds full (see Figure 13-9). Inflation of the bag is evaluated again when establishing appropriate flow to the patient.

G. Place the nasal hood or face mask on the patient (Figure 13-10). Ask the patient to assist you in obtaining a snug but comfortable fit.

  1. Instruct the patient to adjust it at any time throughout the procedure. Allowing patients this option gives them a sense of control.

  2. Adjust the conducting tubes behind the patient's head to ensure a snug fit (see Figure 13-10). This will decrease the amount of air leaking from the mask.

    a. Take care not to tighten the apparatus so that patient movement is prohibited or pressure marks appear on the face.

    b. A piece of gauze may be folded over the patient's nose to minimize gas leakage should adjustment be inadequate.

  3. Not only does an improper fit waste gas, but trace gas leakage contaminates the clinician's immediate environment (breathing zone).

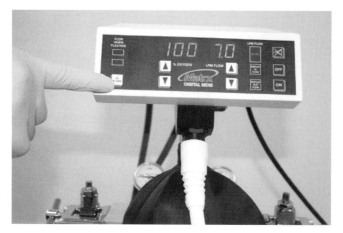

Figure 13-9 Begin the flow of oxygen at an average rate per minute and fill the reservoir bag two-thirds full by use of the O_2 flush button.

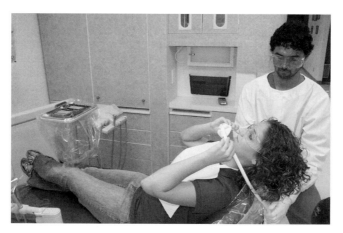

Figure 13-10 Secure the nasal hood to the patient.

H. Determine the appropriate tidal volume needed for the patient by use of the flow of 100% O_2.
　　1. Ask patients if the flow is sufficient to enable them to breathe comfortably. Also determine whether the patient feels that there is gas leaking out of the mask.
　　2. The reservoir bag is a good indicator for appropriate flow[2] (Box 13-1).
　　　　a. If the bag is bulging (Figure 13-11), the patient most likely is not breathing as much gas as is flowing from the machine. The extra gas is being retained in the bag, causing it to overinflate. It is also possible that the patient is mouth-breathing. Often, the breathing pattern becomes more normal and relaxed once the patient becomes familiar with the nasal hood.
　　　　b. Turn down the O_2 level (L/min) until the bag deflates to about two-thirds full.
　　　　c. If the bag continues to inflate like a balloon, it is possible that flow has been blocked somehow (Figure 13-12). Sometimes the bag may get caught between cylinders or the nonrebreathing valve may stick. Attend to this situation quickly.

> **Box 13-1** **DETERMINING APPROPRIATE GAS FLOW IN LITERS PER MINUTE (L/MIN) BEFORE TITRATING N_2O**
>
> • Begin at an average flow of 6–8 L/min O_2 for an adult or 4–6 L/min for a child.
> • If the reservoir bag collapses or flattens, fill it again by use of the O_2 flush valve and increase the flow.
> • If the reservoir bag balloons or overinflates, decrease the flow until the bag is two thirds full.

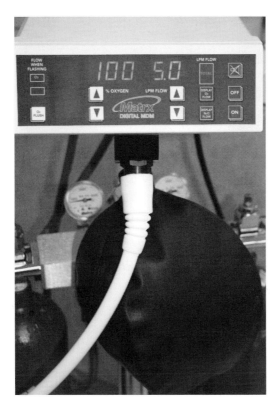

Figure 13-11 Reduce the tidal volume if the reservoir bag is bulging.

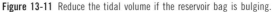

      d. If the bag is collapsing, the patient is breathing all of the flow coming from the machine plus the reserve stored in the reservoir bag. In this case, increase the amount of flow to the patient. It will be necessary to reinflate the reservoir bag by use of the O_2 flush button (Figure 13-13).

I. Once appropriate total liters flow per minute has been established, this amount will remain constant for the duration of the procedure.

IV. ADMINISTRATION OF N_2O

A. Administration technique. Depending on the type of machine, there may be slight variations in the administration technique.

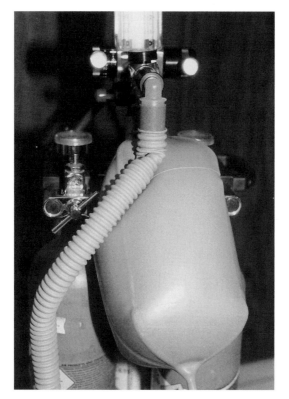

Figure 13-12 Be aware of potential problems, such as kinking hoses.

1. If there are two controls on the machine that independently adjust the levels of each gas, the operator will have to *manually* adjust both the O_2 and the N_2O during administration. Each time N_2O is added, the amount of O_2 will have to be decreased to keep the total liters flow per minute constant.

2. Some machines *automatically* decrease the amount of O_2 whenever N_2O is added to keep the established flow constant.

3. No matter what type of machine is being used, it is important to keep the established liters flow per minute constant throughout the procedure.

    a. On machines that are digital, the LED number displayed indicates the total liters flow per minute.

    b. On machines with dual tubes and floating balls, total liters flow is calculated by adding the numbers from both sides of the flowmeter at the level of the middle of a floating ball. For example, 2 L/min N_2O + 5 L/min O_2 = 7 total liters flow per minute (Figure 13-14).

    c. The number associated with a floating ball does not indicate the percentage of N_2O being delivered. For example, 2 L/min N_2O *does not equal* 20% N_2O.

    d. The actual percentage of N_2O is calculated by dividing the N_2O L/min by the total L/min. For example,

$$\frac{2 \text{ L/min } N_2O}{7 \text{ L/min}} = 28.5\% \text{ N}_2\text{O}$$

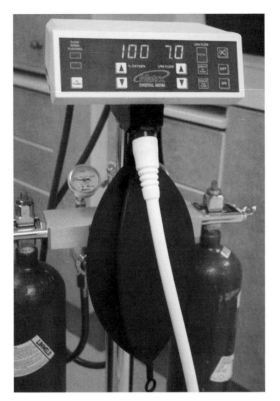

Figure 13-13 Increase the tidal volume if the reservoir bag collapses.

     e. N_2O percentages have been calculated for you and are available for your convenience in Appendix B. They may be photocopied, laminated, and attached to your machine or placed in your operatory.

     f.   On machines that have the percent of O_2 displayed, it is necessary to subtract the number from 100% to obtain the percent of N_2O being delivered. For example, when 60% O_2 is displayed, 40% N_2O is being delivered. Current models also display the percent of nitrous oxide being delivered.

B. *The administration technique of titrating N_2O is recognized as the standard of care* (Box 13-2). Slow titration of small doses of drug is important to prevent oversedation.

C. There is not an exact amount of N_2O that is required to be delivered during the titration technique.

     1. However, a recommended regimen is to begin with approximately 10% to 15% N_2O or 1 to 1.5 L, and add N_2O thereafter in increments with time between each increment (Box 13-3 and Figures 13-15 and 13-16). There is no prescribed amount that must be delivered; rather, it is important to be cognizant of the patient's response. Suggested increments may range from 5% to 10% (0.5–1.0 L).

     2. When beginning to add N_2O, it is preferable to wait at least 60 seconds (1 minute) after a dose before adding the next increment (Figure 13-17).

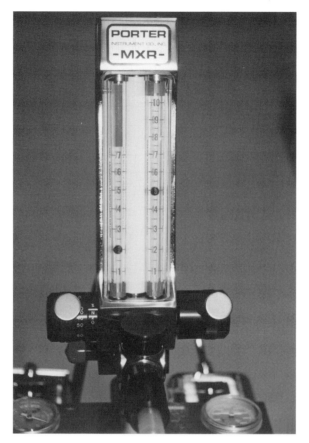

Figure 13-14 Tidal volume is calculated by adding the numbers associated with the height of the balls. *(Courtesy of Porter Instrument Co.)*

3. When sedation is becoming evident, it may be desirable to wait longer between doses. Doses administered too close together with insufficient time in between does not allow for peak effect of one dose to take place before another dose is given.

4. Instruct the patient to breathe through the nose when a nasal hood is used and to keep the lips sealed. This allows for a more accurate level of sedation and gives the clinician a better idea of when an appropriate level is reached. If the patient is talking excessively or verbalizing answers to clinician questioning during administration of N_2O doses, the level of sedation may be altered when the patient resumes nasal breathing. Also, mouth breathing and/or talking are a major source of ambient air contamination.

D. Watch patient comfort level. Titrate to a level of sedation that is determined by patient comfort and relaxation. Watch closely for the signs and symptoms of ideal sedation (Figure 13-18).

1. Remember, there is no preset percentage or fixed dose for N_2O/O_2 sedation for a given patient or experience.

Box 13-2 **N_2O/O_2 ADMINISTRATION TECHNIQUE**

- Assemble and assess armamentarium; open tanks and turn on flowmeter.
- Confirm scavenging devices to be functioning.
- Health history reviewed; vital signs recorded.
- Informed consent obtained.
- Activate O_2 flow; fill reservoir bag approximately two-thirds full by use of O_2 flush valve.
- Secure nasal hood.
- Establish appropriate tidal volume in L/min by observing reservoir bag.
- Begin N_2O titration.
- Assess patient for signs and symptoms of appropriate sedation.
- Titrate N_2O to desired level.
- Perform operative procedures.
- Terminate N_2O flow; administer 5 minutes postoperative 100% O_2.
- Assess recovery.
- Continue postoperative oxygenation if necessary.
- Ensure recovery and dismiss patient.
- Complete sedation record.
- Disinfect and/or sterilize sedation equipment.

Box 13-3 **N_2O/O_2 ADMINISTRATION TECHNIQUE BY USE OF TITRATION**

- Begin with approximately 10%–15% or about 1–1.5 L of N_2O.
- Increase in increments every few minutes until sedation becomes apparent.
- Continue to add N_2O until the desired level of sedation is achieved.

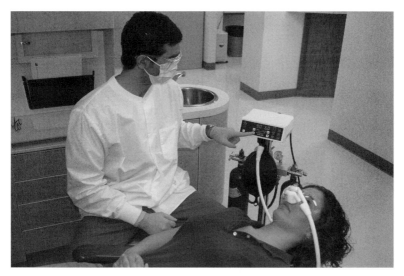

Figure 13-15 Begin titrating 10% to 15% N_2O or approximately 1 to 1.5 L.

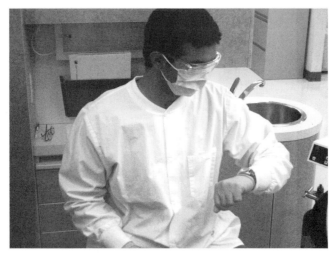

Figure 13-16 The titration techique requires time between increments.

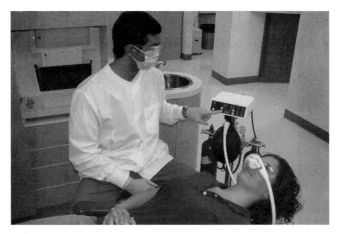

Figure 13-17 Continue adding N_2O until the desired level of sedation is achieved.

2. The percentage of N_2O administered to a patient for a given experience will, most likely, not be the same for any subsequent experience. Individual biovariability accounts for this variation in amount.

E. Intraoperative monitoring includes vigilant observation of the patient's responses and reactions in addition to observation of the reservoir bag.

1. The reservoir bag serves as a monitor of the patient's respirations. The bag inflates and deflates slightly with the patient's inhalations and exhalations. Use this as a sign of depth, rate, and reflection of lung activity.

2. Cumulative effects of N_2O may be seen as the duration of delivery increases. The level of sedation may deepen, resulting in uncomfortable symptoms for the patient. Ask patients periodically how they are feeling.

3. Levels of sedation may be influenced if the patient is allowed to maintain conversation and breathe through the mouth. Therefore, patient talking should be kept to a minimum.
4. If administering concentrations of 50% N_2O or greater, it is advised to refer to the ASA guidelines for additional monitoring procedures.

F. While performing operative procedures (Figure 13-19), the goal is to keep the patient relaxed and comfortable (Figure 13-20).

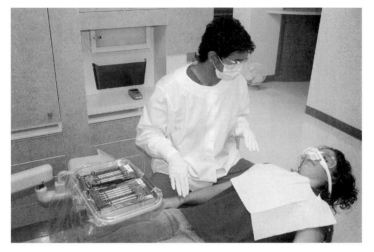

Figure 13-18 Assess the patient for signs and symptoms.

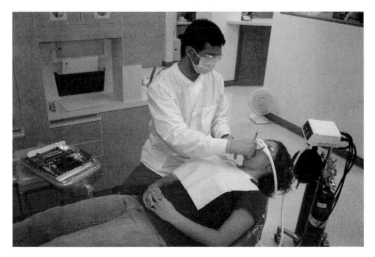

Figure 13-19 Perform procedures when patient is appropriately sedated.

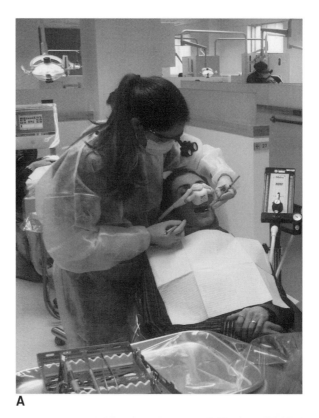

A

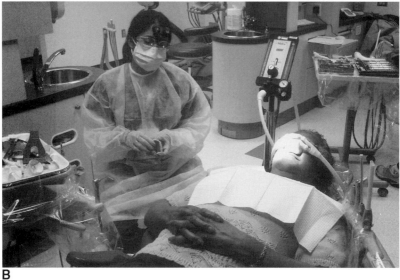

B

Figure 13-20 A and **B**, Perform procedures when the patient is appropriately sedated.

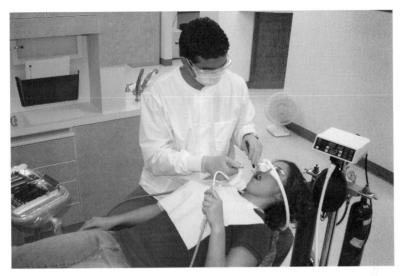

Figure 13-21 Begin postoperative oxygenation (5-minute minimum) near the completion of procedure.

1. Adjust the level of N_2O as needed, depending on the intensity of the procedures and the responses of the patient.
2. You may decrease the N_2O incrementally to a lesser amount for certain nonstimulating phases of treatment and/or completely if you are nearing completion of treatment.

G. When you terminate the N_2O flow, continue delivering 100% O_2 during the final minutes of the operative procedure (Figure 13-21). This begins your required postoperative oxygenation period of 5 minutes minimum. It is vital to pay close attention to this minimum time.
1. It is unnecessary and inappropriate to use the O_2 flush button to remove the admixture of gases from the bag to provide 100% O_2, because this contaminates the environment with N_2O. The technique of lifting the nasal hood off of the patient and purging the contents of the reservoir bag by squeezing it (Figure 13-22) represents an inappropriate technique and is not recommended.[2]
2. To begin the postoperative oxygenation period of 100% O_2, simply terminate the flow of N_2O and continue the flow of O_2.
3. If you administer O_2 for the required time during the final nonintensive phase of the procedure, the patient may be assessed for recovery as soon as the procedure is completed and dismissed rather than having to wait for the postoperative oxygenation period to begin.

H. Assess the recovery of the patient. See Chapter 14 for specific details on recovery procedures.
1. If the patient senses any lethargy, dizziness, light-headedness, or headache, continue 100% O_2 for additional minutes. **Continue 100% O_2 for as long as is necessary** (Figure 13-23).
2. Obtain postoperative vital sign measurements. This can be done during the 5 minutes of postoperative oxygen delivery (Figure 13-24).
3. When, and only when, the patient feels normal, you can remove the breathing apparatus and allow the patient to breathe room air.

I. Extend your appreciation of the patient's cooperation and trust. Reinforce the success of the appointment, then dismiss the patient (Figure 13-25).
J. A condensed version of the administration technique can be found in Appendix E.

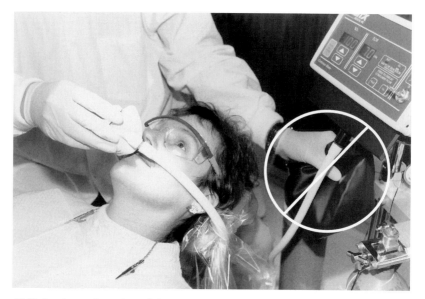

Figure 13-22 Do not purge the contents of the reservoir bag before postoperative oxygenation; this contaminates the operator's breathing zone unnecessarily.

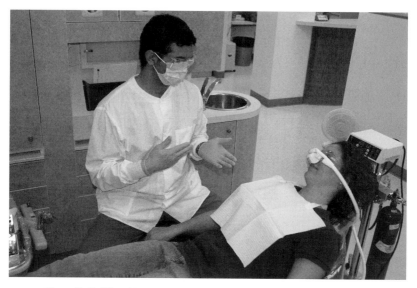

Figure 13-23 Offer additional minutes of oxygen until complete recovery is ensured.

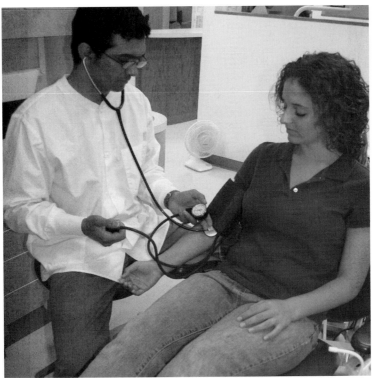

Figure 13-24 Obtain postoperative vital sign measurements to assess recovery.

V. POSTOPERATIVE PROCEDURES

A. It is important to record information regarding the sedation procedure in the patient's file just as you would document delivering local anesthesia or performing an operative procedure. Careful and thorough documentation is necessary for each patient. A later section of this chapter provides details of recordkeeping procedures.

B. Turn off the unit by use of the master switch on the flowmeter.

C. Turn off gas cylinders on a portable unit immediately after use. Central system cylinders are commonly turned off at the end of the day, but lines typically remain charged.

   1. Bleeding the lines on the portable unit at the end of the day purges the gas left in the lines into the room air.

   2. The amount, of gas from bleeding the lines will be minimal; however, it is unnecessary contamination.

VI. STERILIZATION AND DISINFECTION

A. Consult the manufacturer's instructions for best results regarding the sterilization and disinfection of specific sedation equipment.

B. The level of disinfection and/or sterilization depends largely on the piece of equipment itself and its relation to patient contact or the contaminated environment.

   1. As previously mentioned, a clear bag barrier may be placed over the flowmeter as a means of protection against aerosols and splatter. If a bag barrier is not used, surface

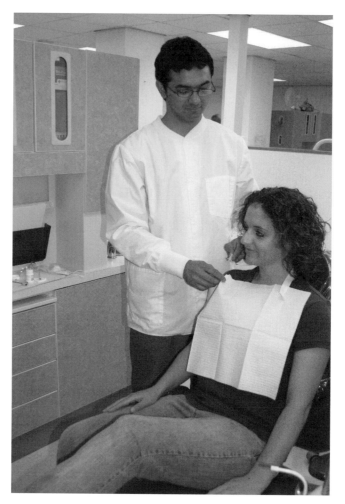

Figure 13-25 Dismiss the patient when recovery is complete.

disinfection may be accomplished by use of a product similar to that used on other operatory surfaces (Figure 13-26).

2. The inside of the reservoir bag is exposed only to fresh gas. Therefore, the inside does not have to be either disinfected or sterilized. However, the outside of the bag may be exposed to aerosols and splatter during operative procedures and should be, at least, disinfected.

   a. Some reservoir bags are autoclavable, whereas others will not stand the rigors of sterilization well. If you choose to sterilize a bag that is not specifically identified as being autoclavable, it is important to know that it will not last very long. A replacement bag should be readily available.

3. The conduction tubing is exposed to both the patient and the environment. No studies verify disease transmission between patients through conduction tubing.

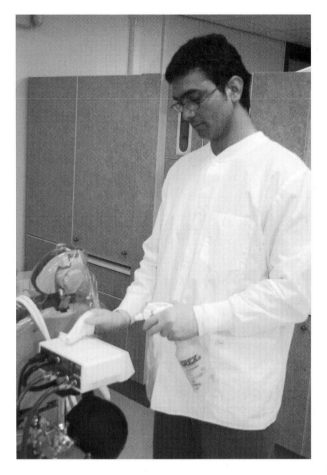

Figure 13-26 Surface disinfection of sedation equipment.

    a. Most of the conduction tubing is able to withstand sterilization. However, if the tubing has a portion that is larger in diameter and corrugated, this piece is not able to withstand heat and will melt. This portion is typically the piece that comes off of the flowmeter and is where the fresh gas first enters the tubing. This section may be disinfected with a surface agent or covered with a barrier.

    b. The other portion of the conduction tubing may be sterilized. If the system has a plastic gauge that monitors the flow of the suction at the end of the hose, this piece may not be sterilized. It may be surface disinfected (Figure 13-27).

4. A laboratory study done in the late 1970s found that nasal bacteria could be transferred into the nasal hood.[3] Two types of nasal hoods are available: sterilizable and single-patient use.

    a. Autoclavable nasal hoods are available from all companies. Sterilization of these products is recommended between patients.

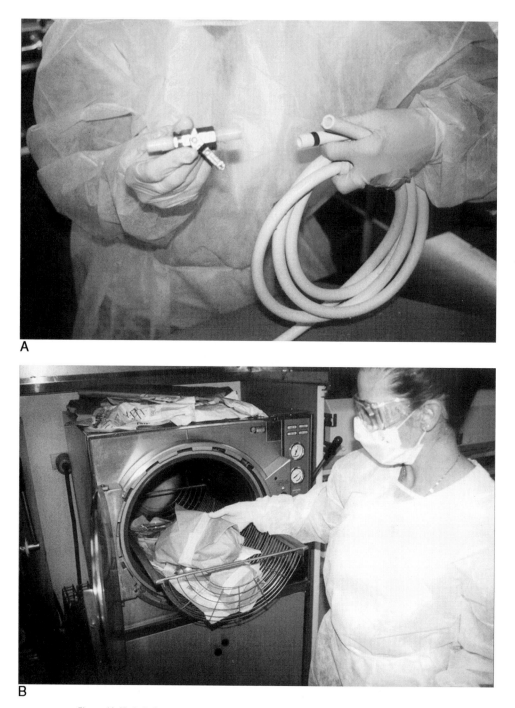

A

B

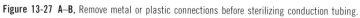

Figure 13-27 A–B, Remove metal or plastic connections before sterilizing conduction tubing.

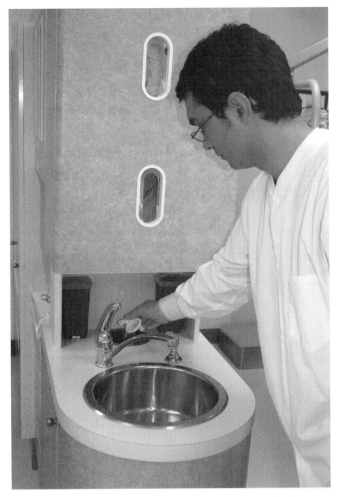

Figure 13-28 Single-patient-use nasal hoods are not autoclavable.

    b. Nasal hoods that are designed for single-patient use are not autoclavable. They may be disposed of (Figure 13-28) or can be retained by the patient or office for a subsequent visit.

VII. RECORDKEEPING PROCEDURES

A. **Importance**
    1. The primary purpose for keeping accurate and complete records in a healthcare setting is to provide a written history of patient–operator interactions. This runs the gamut from the patient's health history, medications, and chief concerns to treatment options, completed procedures, recommendations, and much more.
    2. This history gives an account for future reference to yourself or others so that the patient receives continuity of care.

3. It is also a written record of chronologic events and experiences, making it a medico-legal document able to be used in a court of law.
4. It is recommended that the person making an entry in a patient's record sign or initial the entry. This will hold all individuals accountable for the information, or lack thereof, that is written or unwritten.

B. **Completing the N_2O/O_2 sedation record**
   1. Specific information obtained during N_2O/O_2 sedation should be recorded in the patient's file. This information may be recorded as part of the appointment entry on the patient's service record or on a separate form. Box 13-4 lists the items to include in the patient's file for each experience.
   2. If a separate form is used, it must be permanently attached to the patient's file. A new form is to be used for each experience (Figure 13-29).

Box 13-4 | **COMPONENTS OF THE SEDATION RECORD**

- Patient's name and date
- ASA classification
- Indications for N_2O/O_2 use
- Preoperative, intraoperative, and postoperative vital sign values
- Patient's tidal volume
- Peak percentage of N_2O administered
- Duration of drug administered
- Assessment of recovery (i.e., postoperative oxygenation time in minutes, patient responses to questions)
- Adverse reactions and comments
- Practitioner's signature or initials

N_2O/O_2 Sedation Record

Date: __11-15-08__ Patient Name: __John Doe__ Age: __47__

ASA Classification: (I)   II   III   IV

Indications for N_2O/O_2: __Mild anxiety, hypersensitive gag reflex__

Procedural Data:

	Preoperative	Intraoperative (when >50% N_2O)	Postoperative
Blood pressure:	130/82		126/80
Pulse:	76		72
Respiration:	16		16
SpO_2 (When > 50% N_2O):			

Tidal volume (L/min): __8.0__   Peak % N_2O admin: __40%__

Duration of admin: __35__ min   Postop 100% O_2: __5__ min

Recovery (pt comments): __"Feel fine"__

Adverse Reactions/Comments: __Appt went well__

Clinician's signature: __JJohnson__

Figure 13-29 Sample completed sedation record.

3. There may be items required by state statute or practice act rule that are different from those listed in this reference. Consult the state practice act where you live to determine whether additional items need to be recorded other than those identified.
4. An example of an N_2O/O_2 sedation record can be found in Appendix C. It may be photocopied for office use.

REFERENCES

1. Malamed SF: *Sedation: A Guide to Patient Management,* ed 4, St. Louis, 2003, Mosby.
2. American Dental Association Council on Scientific Affairs: Nitrous oxide in the dental office, *J Am Dent Assoc* 128:364, 1997.
3. Hunt LM, Yagiela JA: Bacterial contamination and transmission by nitrous oxide sedation apparatus, *Oral Surg* 44(3):367, 1977.

Recovery from N₂O/O₂ Sedation

Recovery from N_2O/O_2 sedation is an important part of the sedation experience. Several components of the process are necessary to complete recovery. The literature holds a plethora of references regarding psychological and psychomotor effects that occur during N_2O/O_2 administration.[1-10] The extent of psychological and psychomotor effects during N_2O/O_2 sedation is not the same for any two individuals. Recovery time varies from individual to individual and can depend on a number of factors.[1-10] Return to physiologic normalcy from N_2O/O_2 sedation seems to be readily apparent; however, the prudent practitioner acknowledges the potential for individual biovariability regarding all aspects of recovery and acts with common sense regarding patient dismissal from the clinical setting.

I. PRINCIPLES OF RECOVERY

A. Generally, emergence (recovery) is a mirror image of induction.[11] This mirror image includes patients returning to their original emotional state, as well as recovering from the pharmacologic action of the drug. N_2O provides a rapid onset of clinical signs and thus a correlated rapid emergence will occur. The calm, tranquil induction state should mirror the post-recovery state.

B. Physiologically, recovery occurs the same way for any individual. N_2O, as mentioned earlier, is principally exhaled unchanged from the lungs. However, the potential exists for postoperative symptoms such as lethargy, headache, and nausea to occur. Although opinions vary among researchers as to what causes these symptoms, we believe that postoperative oxygenation is required. Postoperative oxygenation remains an extremely important concept of recovery. Postoperatively, 100% N_2O must be administered for a minimum of 5 minutes. Depending on individual biovariability, this postoperative oxygenation period may be extended until both patient and operator are satisfied that adequate recovery has been achieved.

II. PSYCHOLOGICAL AND PSYCHOMOTOR EFFECTS

A. Investigation of effects. Several studies have been completed by reputable researchers investigating the effects of N_2O on psychomotor ability, memory, mood, and cognition.[1-10] Many tests have been commonly used to assess these functions: visual analog scales have been used to assess mood; psychomotor impairment has been assessed by use of digit-symbol substitution tests, paper-and-pencil tests, eye-hand coordination tests, automobile driving simulation, etc.; and questionnaires have been used to ascertain degrees of euphoria, concentration, and attention. Results of these tests vary; however, there is agreement that mental and psychomotor impairment does occur with N_2O, as it does with almost every other sedative drug.

B. Psychological and psychomotor impairment during N_2O/O_2 administration has been well established. Operators need to be assured to the greatest extent possible that patients are adequately recovered from sedation so they do not harm themselves or others on dismissal from practitioners' offices. To date, there are no references to cases in which patients who were dismissed after N_2O/O_2 sedation harmed or injured themselves or others because of incomplete recovery.

III. TECHNIQUE FOR ASSESSING ADEQUATE RECOVERY

A. Patient escorts. Depending on the circumstances of the situation, a practitioner must dismiss treatment based on knowledge of the drug effects and the patient's response. Following N_2O/O_2 sedation, a fully recovered patient does not need an escort.

B. Assessment of a patient's response to questioning is subjective but in most cases valid.

   1. After the required postoperative oxygenation period of 5 minutes minimum, you should begin questioning patients about how they feel before removing the nasal hood. Patients should indicate that they are feeling fine and not drowsy, light-headed, groggy, dizzy, nauseous, etc. (Figure 14-1).

   2. If there is any indication that a patient does not feel normal, assume that recovery is not complete. Additional postoperative oxygen time is required and continued until all responses are positive and indicative of normal feelings (Box 14-1).

   3. Generally, patients should be alert with a pleasant or happy demeanor (Figures 14-2 and 14-3).

C. Postoperative vital sign values are an objective measure of recovery.

   1. Generally, blood pressure values within 10 mm Hg (both systolic and diastolic) from preoperative readings are considered to be within an accepted comparable range.

   2. Likewise, postoperative pulse rate within 10 beats and respiration rate within 5 breaths are acceptable parameters for comparison (see Figure 14-4).

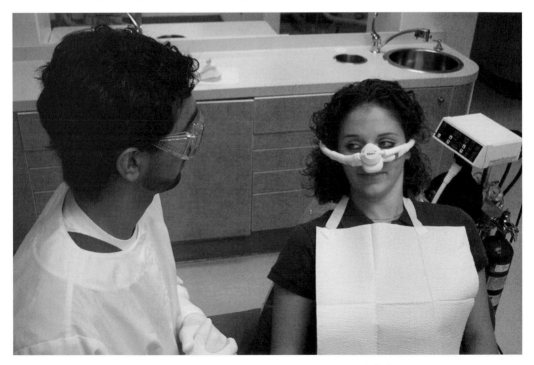

Figure 14-1 Ask the patient questions about how he or she is feeling.

Box 14-1	**ASSESSING RECOVERY**

Assessment begins after initial 5-minute postoperative oxygenation period.
- Obtain postoperative vital sign values.
- Question patient without removing O_2 for indications of:
  - Lethargy
  - Headache
  - Dizziness
  - Confusion
  - Nausea
- If any symptoms present, continue O_2.
- Dismiss only when assured patient is fully recovered.

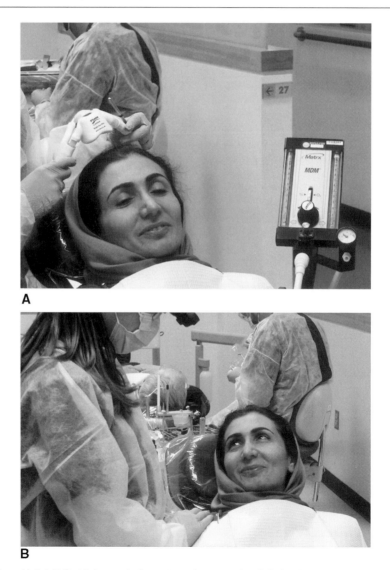

A

B

Figure 14-2 A, Patient feels normal after postoperative oxygenation. **B,** Patient is not groggy or lethargic.

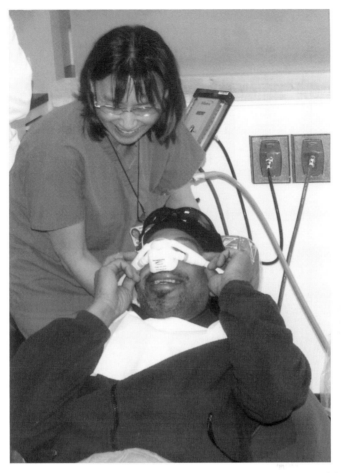

Figure 14-3 Patient feels happy and relaxed after postoperative oxygenation as the nasal hood is removed.

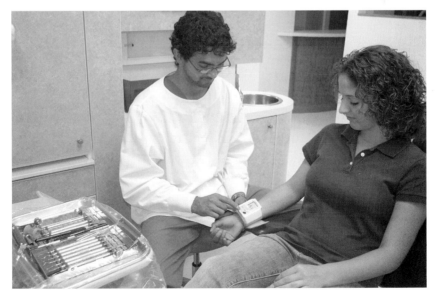

Figure 14-4 Obtain postoperative vital signs to assist assessment of recovery.

D. Psychomotor recovery from inhalation sedation has been addressed in the literature.

    1. Early studies[12–14] recommended preoperative and postoperative drawing tests to determine visuomotor coordination and recovery. In the studies, recovery was complete within 3–5 minutes after termination of the N_2O.[12–14]

    2. Jastak and Orendurff[15] investigated psychomotor recovery by use of a driving simulation test. Participants were evaluated for errors in steering, braking, signaling, and speeding. All postsedation figures correlated with presedation values, thereby concluding that patients could safely operate a motor vehicle after N_2O/O_2 sedation.[15] This study has been the foundation for practitioners dismissing patients without an escort. Recently, Martin *et al*[16] confirmed the claim that driving ability is not impaired after flexible sigmoidoscopy screening with N_2O.

    3. There is a simple hand-eye coordination exercise that can be done in the office to assess psychomotor recovery. Have patients extend an arm in front of them; then give instructions to place one of their fingers on the tip of their nose. The exercise may be

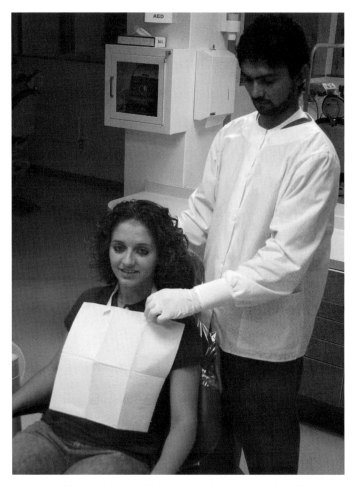

Figure 14-5 Dismiss the patient only when adequate recovery is achieved.

done with either or both hands. Accuracy is subjective; however, if this simple skill cannot be completed, it may be necessary to reevaluate adequate recovery. It is important to only verbalize without demonstrating this technique as cognitive recognition becomes part of the assessment of recovery.

IV. ADEQUATE RECOVERY

A. Patients should be alert and oriented.

B. Vital sign values should be stable and within acceptable limits.

C. Use of scoring systems may assist in documentation of fitness for discharge. The Vancouver Sedative Recovery Scale has been cited as a valid assessment tool for assessing recovery after sedation.[17] Twelve items of observation are divided into three broad categories: response, eye appearance and function, and body movement.[17]

D. Documentation of adequate recovery must be maintained for each patient visit.[18] It is important to record that 100% O_2 was administered postoperatively and to note the length of time that it was given.

V. RECOVERY TIME

A. Recovery time has continued to be a subject of research studies through the years. A wide variety of recommendations exist regarding the number of minutes it takes for complete recovery after sedation with N_2O. The important factor to remember is that each patient is different and recovery times may vary.[19-21] Ultimately, responsibility lies in the hands of the clinician to make a decision as to the complete recovery of patients before their dismissal (Figure 14-5).

REFERENCES

1. Cheam EW *et al*: The effect of nitrous oxide on the performance of psychomotor tests: a dose-response study, *Anaesthesia* 50:764, 1995.
2. Fagan D *et al*: A dose-response study of the effects of inhaled nitrous oxide on psychological performance and mood, *Psychopharmacology* 116:333, 1994.
3. Dohrn CS *et al*: Subjective and psychomotor effects of nitrous oxide in healthy volunteers, *Behav Pharmacol* 3:19, 1992.
4. Armstrong PJ *et al*: Effects of nitrous oxide on psychological performance: a dose-response study using inhalation of concentrations up to 15%, *Psychopharmacology* 117:486, 1995.
5. Zacny JP *et al*: Time course of effects of brief inhalations of nitrous oxide in normal volunteers, *Addiction* 89:831, 1994.
6. Zacny JP *et al*: The subjective, behavioral and cognitive effects of subanesthetic concentrations of isoflurane and nitrous oxide in healthy volunteers, *Psychopharmacology* 114:409, 1994.
7. Yajnik S *et al*: Effects of marijuana history on the subjective, psychomotor, and reinforcing effects of nitrous oxide in humans, *Drug Alcohol Depend* 36:227, 1994.
8. Tiplady R, Sinclair WA, Morrison LM: Effects of nitrous oxide on psychological performance, *Psychopharmacol Bull* 28:207, 1992.
9. Ramsay JS *et al*: Paradoxical effects of nitrous oxide on human memory, *Psychopharmacology* 106:370, 1992.
10. Thompson JM *et al*: Cognitive properties of sedation agents: comparison of the effects of nitrous oxide and midazolam on memory and mood, *Br Dent J* 187(10):557, 1999.
11. Eger EI II: Uptake and distribution. In Miller RD, editor. *Anesthesia*, vol 1, ed 4, New York, 1994, Churchill Livingstone.
12. Newman MG, Trieger N, Miller JC: Measuring recovery from anesthesia: a simple test, *Anesth Anal* 48:136, 1969.
13. Trieger N, Newman MG, Miller JC: An objective measure of recovery, *Anesth Prog* 16:4, 1969.
14. Trieger N *et al*: Nitrous oxide: a study of physiological and psychomotor effects, *JADA* 82:142, 1971.

15. Jastak JT, Orendurff D: Recovery from nitrous sedation, *Anesth Prog* 22:113, 1975.

16. Martin JP *et al*: Inhaled patient-administered nitrous oxide/oxygen mixture does not impair driving ability when used as analgesia during screening flexible sigmoidoscopy, *Gastrointest Endosc* 51(6):701, 2000.

17. Macnab AJ *et al*: A research tool for measurement of recovery from sedation: the Vancouver Sedative Recovery Scale, *J Ped Surg* 26(11):1263, 1991.

18. American Dental Association: *Guidelines for the Use of Conscious Sedation, Deep Sedation and General Anesthesia for Dentists*, Chicago, 2002, American Dental Association.

19. McKercher TC *et al*: Recovery and enhancement of reflex reaction time after nitrous oxide analgesia, *JADA* 101:785, 1980.

20. Korttila K *et al*: Time course of mental and psychomotor effects of 30 percent nitrous oxide during inhalation and recovery, *Anesthesiology* 54:220, 1981.

21. Trojan J *et al*: Immediate recovery of psychomotor function after patient-administered nitrous oxide/oxygen inhalation for colonoscopy, *Endoscopy* 29:17, 1997.

Chapter 15

Multidisciplinary Application of N_2O/O_2 Sedation

Some health disciplines have been using N_2O/O_2 sedation for mild-to-moderate pain control and anxiety relief for many years. Other healthcare professionals have recently revisited its use, not as a general anesthetic but as an effective analgesic-sedative for the many ambulatory and outpatient procedures being performed today.

Articles referring to N_2O/O_2 sedation in obstetrics are found in the literature because of long-standing use in Great Britain.[1] Emergency care personnel, in both the field and the hospital setting, have also been long-term providers of this therapy.[2] Other disciplines have limited literature citations.

N_2O may have broad applicability in an era in which greater numbers of surgical procedures are being performed in outpatient settings. N_2O/O_2 sedation is a viable treatment alternative for outpatient procedures in a variety of disciplines.

I. EMERGENCY MEDICINE

A. Prehospital care in the ambulance

1. An analgesic agent appropriate for prehospital emergency pain control should possess several specific characteristics. Properties that are desirable are rapid onset of clinical action, no effect on level of consciousness, no significant side effects, and no masking of other conditions, which would ultimately interfere with the diagnostic evaluation at the hospital.

2. N_2O possesses most of these characteristics. Several researchers support the notion that N_2O possesses many of the ideal characteristics necessary in this discipline.[3–5]

3. Historical use of N_2O/O_2 in emergency medicine. The first self-administered, fixed-ratio system used in an ambulance service was implemented by Peter Baskett, from England, in 1969. A mixture of 50% N_2O and 50% O_2 was delivered to the patient by use of an on-demand system. His idea was that patients in an ambulatory situation should control their own sedation by self-administering this fixed-ratio mixture of gases. Baskett concluded his clinical trials (305 patients with significant decrease in pain and no serious complications) with the claim that N_2O/O_2 was safe and effective for use in emergency medicine.[2]

4. Current usage and effectiveness statistics

   a. Recently emergency medical services (EMS) have placed priority on early patient stabilization, safe transportation, and effective communication systems (Figure 15-1). Great strides have been made in these areas, making services to the public safer and more effective. Pain control has always been a focus and is gaining greater attention. The issues of masking symptoms or making conditions worse before hospital access are important considerations in the decision to attend to pain with an analgesic agent.

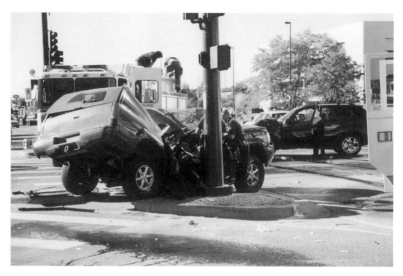

Figure 15-1 First responders at the scene.

    b. EMS personnel continue to use Baskett's fixed-ratio, self-administration technique. This technique is popular because of its portability in the field. Emergency departments in hospital settings may use the fixed-ratio, on-demand equipment, or they may use continuous-flow machines like those that have been used in dentistry.

    c. Faddy and Garlick completed a systematic review of the literature regarding prehospital treatment of patients with a 50%/50% N_2O and O_2 mixture.[6] Their review analyzed adverse events, recovery time, and need for additional medication.[6] They concluded that because of a low incidence of reported adverse events, N_2O and O_2 could be safely administered by lay responders.[6]

B. **Use in hospital emergency departments**

    1. Not long after the initiation of prehospital sedation in England, healthcare providers in the United States began to use it for emergency medicine in the hospital. In 1979, Flomenbaum *et al*[7] were the first to promote its use in U.S. emergency departments and to document such use in the literature.

    2. Researchers have cited many instances of successful uses of N_2O/O_2 in emergency department settings.[3–5,8,9] Gamis *et al*[10] completed a study that used N_2O/O_2 on pediatric patients requiring laceration repair in the emergency department at Children's Mercy Hospital in Kansas City, Missouri. Thirty-four children participated and were placed in either a treatment group that used a ratio of 30% N_2O and 70% O_2 or a control group that used 100% O_2. A clinically significant difference was found in the pain scores between groups of children older than 8 years. Although no statistically significant difference was found with children in the 2–7 age group, pain scores decreased when N_2O/O_2 was used.[10] In other studies, N_2O/O_2 provided a significant reduction in pain and anxiety during venous cannulation in the emergency department.[11,12]

    3. White *et al*[13] recently confirmed that prehospital pain control can be improved, especially for patients with extremity fractures. They acknowledge N_2O as a viable option. Orthopedic fracture care in the emergency department of a hospital has also had success with nitrous oxide and oxygen.[14,15]

4. When providing patient care of the skin, N_2O/O_2 may be used when placing and removing sutures; incising abscesses; removing cysts, nevi, or warts; débriding wounds; and dressing burns.

5. Head injuries that are nonneurologic in origin may be successfully treated with N_2O/O_2. Examples are abrasion débridement, removing or draining abscesses or cysts, removing foreign objects from ears, and removing or replacing teeth after trauma.

6. Examples of other procedures include removing or changing drains, catheterization, biopsies, splinting, extrications, complicated transfer or movement of patients, and other musculoskeletal injuries, including strains, sprains, and dislocations.

C. Contraindications for use of N_2O/O_2 in emergency medicine

1. In emergency cases in which pneumothorax or a closed head injury is suspected, N_2O is not recommended.[10]

D. Equipment

1. The equipment used in ambulances consists of the gas mixture stored in either a single cylinder or in separate tanks. In some countries, the single-cylinder system is preferred because it is lightweight and easy to operate. A major disadvantage of this 50:50 mixture is the instability of the gases in one cylinder. If the temperature of the mixture is allowed to fall below 5.5° C for even a limited amount of time, the N_2O separates and settles to the bottom of the cylinder. A high concentration of O_2 could be dispensed under these conditions, which would mean that pure N_2O would be dispensed as the O_2 is depleted.

2. To date, the United States has not approved the single-cylinder system for use because of the potential for 100% N_2O to be delivered. However, this system is popular in countries such as the United Kingdom, Canada, Australia, and New Zealand.

3. Matrx by Midmark offers the safety of a double-tank system and the portability of the single-cylinder system. Its major advantage is that it weighs only 11 lb and can be carried over the shoulder or harnessed to the back. The Nitronox field model is shown in Figure 15-2.

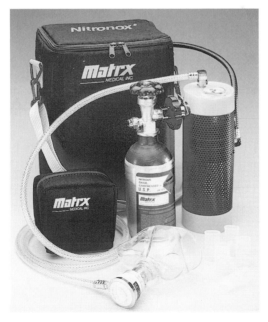

Figure 15-2 Nitronox field model. *(Courtesy of Henry Schein.)*

4. In the field setting, patients are required to hold a mask and place it over their mouth and nose to inspire the gas. If the patient is unable to hold the mask because of an injury, a mouthpiece can be held tight between the lips and teeth, allowing for inspiration through the mouth.

E. Products
1. The 50:50 gas mixture that is primarily used in the United Kingdom, Canada, and Australia is called Entonox. It is manufactured by several companies.
2. Nitronox is available both in the United States and abroad.

II. OBSTETRICS AND GYNECOLOGY

A. Labor and delivery
1. The literature is saturated with studies reporting manageable, successful labor and deliveries with N_2O/O_2 therapy.
2. A Russian physician began the use of N_2O/O_2 in 1880 as an analgesic during labor. His experiments led him to the conclusion that it relieved labor pain without harming mother or baby.[16]
3. Swedish literature citations confirm the safety record of N_2O anesthesia. Records show no reproductive problems in nearly 300 women exposed to N_2O.[17]
4. A 1981 hospital study in Wales evaluated the effectiveness of Entonox delivered through a nasal catheter to women in labor. Both midwives and mothers agreed that Entonox provided labor pain relief.[18] Administration by nasal catheter was comfortable and nonintrusive; however, this method of delivery should not be used because of environmental contamination.
5. A 1994 study in Toronto done by Carstoniu *et al*[19] raised questions about the validity and reliability of previous research on N_2O/O_2 use in labor, citing methodologic flaws as the primary weakness of early research. In the study, relief of pain and oxygen saturation were the foci. Results showed no statistical difference when patients used N_2O/O_2 or compressed air. Patients did recognize the difference in gases, and when offered to continue either, they preferred N_2O/O_2. The oxygen desaturation factor was insignificant, and authors indicated O_2 levels were enhanced between contractions.[19] However, Fortescue and Wee[20] offered that distraction, relaxation, and control may be reasons why the other researchers did not get statistical significance between nitrous oxide and air.
6. Vallejo *et al*[21] reported 40% nitrous oxide was effective in anxiety reduction during cesarean section at the time of injection and incisions.

B. Gynecologic laparoscopy
1. Although CO_2 is used traditionally as the insufflation gas for laparoscopy, N_2O may be used as part of a combination technique.
2. The American Association of Gynecologic Laparoscopists[22] stated that no adverse incidents occurred in more than 20,000 procedures when N_2O/O_2 was used in some capacity.

III. DERMATOLOGY

A. Hair transplantation
1. Hair transplantation is cited as a procedure in which N_2O/O_2 can provide satisfactory analgesia without negatively affecting patient cooperation or producing untoward side effects. Patients in a study by Sadick and Militana[23] responded overwhelmingly (94%) that they preferred N_2O/O_2 over 10 mg diazepam (Valium) and the Dermajet method

of lidocaine delivery. Because this surgery requires repeated injections of local anesthetic, the analgesic/sedative nature of N_2O/O_2 allows for increased patient tolerance.
2. An N_2O/O_2 advantage noted in hair transplantation is the rapid elimination of the drug versus others, such as diazepam, which has a much longer latent period without reversal.[23]

B. Skin treatments and cancer surgeries. Chemical peeling and skin cancer surgeries are also mentioned in the literature as being facilitated by N_2O/O_2 sedation.[23,24]

C. Liposuction
1. Liposuction has become a popular procedure. Local anesthetic infiltration has been combined with IM, IV, inhalation sedation, or general anesthesia for this procedure. Professionals state that although many drugs interact with local anesthetics required by this procedure, N_2O/O_2 does not.
2. Dermatologists' experience with N_2O/O_2 is minimal; however, they support its adjunctive properties to local anesthetics.[25] Maloney *et al*[26] concur with others in the dermatology field who support the use of N_2O/O_2. In their study, 46 of 47 patients indicated that they would request N_2O/O_2 for future visits and thought it should be used more in the discipline.[26]

IV. PODIATRY

A. Ambulatory foot surgeries
1. Ambulatory foot surgery was successfully accomplished in 1966 with N_2O/O_2 sedation. It was the first mention in the literature of N_2O/O_2 use in this discipline.[27]

B. Various other podiatric procedures
1. In a 1972 study, Mosher and Sorkin[28] provided descriptive evidence of 21 patients requiring varying podiatric procedures while receiving N_2O/O_2 titrated to appropriate levels. No significant side effects were noted; amnesia was reported in 19% of patients. All patients indicated a relaxed sense of well-being. Several advantages of N_2O/O_2 analgesia were listed, one of which was the enhancement of local anesthetic effects.
2. Some of the procedures reported being performed with N_2O/O_2 are digital arthroplasty, nail matricectomy, subungual exostosectomy, bunionectomy, excision of digital mass, digital arthrodesis, excision of hallux ossicle, tailor's bunionectomy, and excision of plantar mass.[28]

C. Use with diazepam (Valium)
Another study (1982) encouraged specialists to use N_2O/O_2 with 10 mg of diazepam. The authors stated success in more than 150 cases. Their attitude regarding this technique is professed as "a new era in the attainment of near-painless podiatric surgery."[29]

V. OPHTHALMOLOGY

A. Eye surgery
1. The most common anesthetic techniques involve IV sedation and retrobulbar block or topical anesthesia only. Cataract surgery with N_2O/O_2 sedation is referenced in the journal *Ophthalmic Surgery*.[30]
2. N_2O/O_2 can be used instead of IM premedication to prepare patients for the necessary local anesthetic placement. McMahan[30] used N_2O/O_2 therapy on 800 patients for cataract surgery with great success.

B. Implant surgery
1. Implant surgery performed at the Hawaiian Eye Surgicenter includes N_2O/O_2 as part of the procedure. Clinicians there wanted an analgesic-sedative for assistance during

the local injection but did not want the prolonged effects of other drugs. They wanted patients to be fully recovered for prompt dismissal.

2. Clinicians expressed satisfaction with the calming, amnestic effects with their 50% N_2O and 50% O_2 technique.[31]

C. Ambulatory setting. Specialists in the ophthalmology discipline acknowledge interest in the use of N_2O/O_2 sedation in the ambulatory setting.[32]

VI. CRYOSURGERY

A. In cryosurgery, N_2O is used to cool metal instruments, which in turn initiates the freezing or tissue necrosis of a lesion.

B. N_2O is preferred over liquid nitrogen because it is easier to handle.[33]

C. Successful management of obstructive malignant airway lesions and early superficial lung cancer with bronchoscopic cryotherapy was shown by Noppen *et al*[34] in Belgium.

VII. PSYCHIATRY AND PSYCHOLOGY

A. Depression
1. N_2O/O_2 has been used for patients exhibiting chronic anxiety. Depressed patients have found relief from N_2O/O_2 therapy.
2. In an early study, N_2O was found to be more effective than thiopental with electroconvulsive therapy for treatment of depression.[35] However, methohexital or propofol plus succinylcholine is still the most commonly used.

B. Schizophrenia
1. Traditionally, the use of N_2O/O_2 with schizophrenic patients has been cautioned because of individual biovariability and the potential for provoking their psychoses.
2. Gillman[36] found three of four patients became relaxed after N_2O/O_2 use. He documented problems with one patient.

C. Sex research
1. Sex research has included N_2O/O_2 therapy as well. Research done by Gillman and Lichtigfeld[37] shows females unable to achieve orgasm became multiorgasmic with therapy that included N_2O/O_2.

D. Hyperactivity
1. deWet *et al*[38] have also used N_2O as a possible treatment modality for hyperactivity. They report a 50% positive response rate and intend to continue with further controlled studies.

E. Additional information
1. N_2O/O_2 sedation use with mentally ill patients requires extreme caution and medical consultation.

VIII. ENDOSCOPY

A. Gastrointestinal endoscopy
1. Diehl *et al*[39] presented N_2O/O_2 research results at the American Society of Gastrointestinal Endoscopy (ASGE) 1996 annual session. They indicated success with N_2O/O_2 in the outpatient setting at significantly less cost. In addition, patients generally accepted the procedure, and clinicians believed that administering N_2O/O_2 was not problematic and appreciated patient tolerance. The study also looked at differences between the use

of N_2O/O_2 or IV-infused barbiturates. No statistically significant differences were found.[39]

B. **Colonoscopy**
1. Forbes reported that the 50%/50% N_2O/O_2 mixture was acceptable for many patients undergoing colonoscopy.[40] They concluded that this may be a viable option for some patients and reported the advantage of faster recovery. Theodorou *et al* agreed as they compared total IV sedation with N_2O/O_2 and sevoflurane inhalation sedation.[41]

C. **Flexible sigmoidoscopy**
1. Flexible sigmoidoscopy has generally been performed in an outpatient setting without anesthesia in the United Kingdom. A placebo-controlled study done by Harding concluded that N_2O and O_2 were beneficial in attenuating patient discomfort during this procedure.[42]

D. **Bronchoscopy**
1. It was determined that N_2O and O_2 could be combined with local anesthesia and be an effective and safe method to perform fiberoptic bronchoscopy for children.[43]

IX. ADDICTION WITHDRAWL

A. **Pentazocine (Talwin)**
1. N_2O has been investigated as a potential therapeutic drug for addiction withdrawal of certain substances. Kripke and Hechtman[44] were the first to mention this innovation in 1972 when treating pentazocine addiction. Pentazocine is a narcotic-analog analgesic. It is contraindicated for treating patients who use narcotics.
2. Pentazocine was used in significant amounts to obviate the continual severe pain of an esophageal (potash) injury plaguing a 14-year-old girl. The patient became addicted to the drug, and clinicians used N_2O/O_2 to wean her from it. Advantages of this therapy were the freedom from pain and the ease of delivery at her home.[44]

B. **Alcohol**
1. Lichtigfeld and Gillman[45] found N_2O/O_2 to be effective for alcohol withdrawal in more than 5000 cases in South Africa.
2. A single 20-minute application of analgesic N_2O/O_2 to a patient during admittance to a treatment center relieves initial withdrawal symptoms without causing significant sedation, which allows for other social detoxification therapies to be initiated immediately.[45] Gillman and Lichtigfeld[46] reported 90% of acute alcoholic withdrawal states were reversed within the first 60 minutes of a single-dose treatment of N_2O/O_2. Other discoveries made with N_2O/O_2 included reduced hospital stays and decreased doses of other medications with no addictive propensity to N_2O.[47]

C. Nicotine and marijuana addiction. N_2O/O_2 sedation has also been experimented with successfully in treating nicotine and marijuana addiction.[47]

X. RADIOLOGY

A. **Painful procedures**
1. Analgesic-anxiolytic N_2O/O_2 has proved beneficial in the discipline of radiology.
2. In a study on radiologic procedures, 50 of 53 patients reported that N_2O/O_2 sedation improved their procedures. Some of the procedures in which N_2O/O_2 sedation may be appropriate are aortoperipheral arteriography, percutaneous biopsy, visceral arteriography, percutaneous cholangiography, biliary catheter placement, biliary stone retrieval,

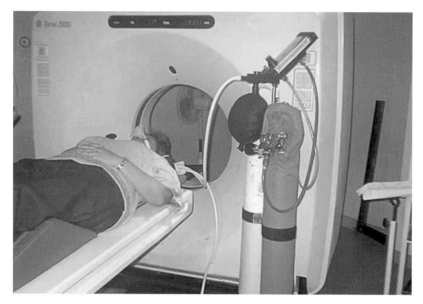

Figure 15-3 N_2O/O_2 administration during a radiologic procedure. *(Photo courtesy of Dr. Carlos Plateroti, Buenos Aires, Argentina.)*

bilateral ureter stent placement, hepatic artery catheter placement, liver abscess drainage, and bilateral temporomandibular joint arthroscopy.[48] Patients who use N_2O/O_2 sedation are far more cooperative when asked to remain still than patients who use IV sedation.[48]

B. **Magnetic resonance imaging (MRI)**
   1. The MRI procedure is often complicated or even contraindicated for patients who are claustrophobic. The procedure requires the patient to be confined to a small space and remain very still for an extended period.
   2. Often patients require some type of sedation for anxiety management so that accuracy of the procedure is ensured. N_2O/O_2 sedation can be a viable option for this procedure. However, it may be necessary to explore ways to improve the accessibility of the delivery equipment within the spatial confines of the MRI equipment (Figure 15-3).

XI. DENTISTRY

A. **Pain and anxiety**
   1. Although N_2O revolutionized pain control in dentistry, local anesthesia is the backbone of today's practice. N_2O/O_2 is often used in tandem with local anesthesia, especially in those patients who have difficulty with needles.
   2. Pain and fear are prohibiting factors for seeking dental treatment; more than 40% of the population avoids the dental office for these reasons.[49] N_2O/O_2 sedation offers a way to overcome these barriers.

B. **Widespread use in the discipline**
   1. Dentistry has been and continues to be a significant supporter and proprietor of N_2O/O_2 sedation. It has been used for most procedures and by all specialties within the profession.
   2. The dental profession uses N_2O/O_2 sedation for procedures in the areas of periodontics, prosthodontics, orthodontics, dental hygiene, restorative dentistry, oral and maxillofacial surgery, endodontics, geriatrics, and especially pedodontics.[50]

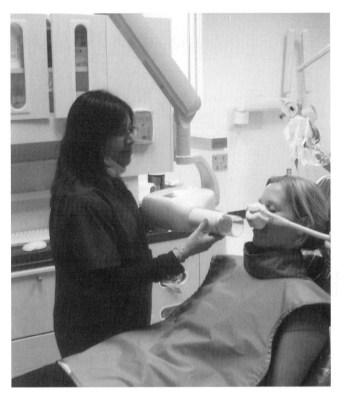

Figure 15-4 Depression of the gag reflex.

C. Depression of the gag reflex (Figure 15-4). Recent studies document that N_2O/O_2 sedation works well to depress a hypersensitive gag reflex, which can be problematic during dental procedures.[51,52]

XII. PEDIATRICS

A. Painful and anxiety-producing situations

1. Pediatric patients present special concerns for healthcare professionals. The more positive healthcare experiences children have, the more likely that they will behave positively during future visits. Also, repeated positive childhood experiences create positive adult attitudes and behaviors. Think of the number of adult patients who are anxious because of a bad childhood experience.

2. Despite a trusting, caring, and kind relationship between a healthcare worker and a child, some procedures hurt. No matter how the clinician prepares children psychologically for pain, the actual stick with the needle is what they remember. In dentistry, N_2O/O_2 sedation of children has been successful for many years. It is estimated that 88% of pediatric dentists use this method of sedation in their practices.[53]

3. Over a 9-year period, Griffin *et al*[54] researched the effect of N_2O/O_2 sedation on more than 3000 children and teenagers for minor surgical procedures. The procedures included laceration or fracture repair, nevi excision, wart removal, abscess incision, and removal

of items such as slivers, needles, nails, and fishhooks. Ninety-nine percent of the patients indicated that they would choose to have N_2O/O_2 sedation at a future visit.

B. Amnestic and hypnosuggestive properties

1. These properties are advantageous when treating children. The short attention span of a child often requires additional patient management and time when completing a procedure. The relaxed patient and altered perception of time offered by N_2O/O_2 sedation greatly assist the practitioner.

2. Children are much more hypnosuggestive than adults. A calm, slow, soothing voice facilitates the action of N_2O/O_2 immensely. See Chapter 16 for information specific to pediatrics.

XIII. ACUTE MYOCARDIAL INFARCTION

A. Reduced pain and anxiety

1. Analgesic levels of N_2O/O_2 have been successfully implemented to relieve acute pain during myocardial infarction (MI). The pathophysiologic process of an MI results in extreme pain and typically includes tremendous anxiety.

2. Several studies conducted from 1962–1965 in the former Soviet Republic proved the effectiveness of N_2O/O_2 with MI.[55,56] Its use in the United States at that time is documented in the literature as well.[9,57] Results of research by Thompson and Lown[58] indicate some relief of pain in 74% of patients. Patients with mild pain were more likely to get more significant relief than those experiencing moderate-to-agonizing pain. In those cases, narcotics provided adjuvant analgesic therapy.[58]

3. Currently, the most common pain relief protocols for acute MI include Nitonox, Entonox, nitroglycerin, beta-blockers, and morphine.

B. Supplemental oxygen

1. N_2O/O_2 proved beneficial for those patients being treated in an ambulatory setting for coronary artery disease by enriching the O_2 supply to the heart.[4]

2. O_2 is critical for perfusion to the myocardium, while the N_2O works as the analgesic-sedative for the patient.[4,13,58]

XIV. TERMINALLY ILL PATIENTS

A. Cancer or terminal illness

1. Children with cancer who must undergo lumbar puncture and bone marrow aspiration reacted favorably to a nitrous oxide/oxygen and midazolam combination used for pain relief during these procedures.[59]

2. Patients with cancer or in terminal stages of illness often have unbearable pain.[60]

3. In such cases, the issue of adequate pain control is a primary focus of the patient's family and significant others. They want their loved one to be comfortable in the final stages of life or when suffering a debilitating illness.

B. Quality of life

1. Fosburg and Crone[61] reported that some patients continue IV-infused narcotics in conjunction with N_2O/O_2 treatment, whereas others prefer N_2O/O_2 alone. Keating and Kundrat[62] reported that 81% of N_2O treatments provided improvement in pain that lasted from 30 minutes to 2 hours. In addition, they reported increased activity, smiling, and communicability in patients.

2. Patients may be treated at home with N_2O/O_2 therapy and can often control their own therapy. In many instances of terminal illness, the N_2O/O_2 therapy improved patients' moods and appetites, and patients communicated more freely.

C. **Hemodynamics**
1. The hemodynamic issues surrounding continuous, long-term use of N_2O/O_2 are obviously not as important as relief of pain and anxiety for these patients in the final stages of life.
2. Again, patient comfort is a top priority; restful, relaxed, pain-free last days are intensely sought by all terminally ill patients.

XV. MISCELLANEOUS PROCEDURES

A. Gillman and Lichtigfeld[47] cited that symptoms associated with various neurologic disorders have been eliminated with the use of N_2O/O_2 sedation. Some examples are Tourette's syndrome, neuroleptic-induced akathisia, and spasmodic torticollis. The article refers to these as preliminary investigations that require specific organized study.[47]
B. N_2O was shown to be an effective analgesic for patients undergoing percutaneous liver biopsy. Pain scores were significantly lower for patients in the N_2O/O_2 treatment group versus patients treated with a placebo. Investigators in this study cited several favorable characteristics of N_2O in addition to its analgesic potential.[63]
C. Migraine headaches have been treated with analgesic concentrations of N_2O/O_2. It seems the analgesic and sedative properties of N_2O/O_2 assist with the management of migraine symptoms.
1. In the literature, a 30-minute treatment of N_2O/O_2 titrated specifically to the patient's needs brought total relief within that period.[64] A more recent study validates this claim and indicates 80% of 22 patients with acute migraine symptoms who came to the emergency department did not require rescue medication after treatment with N_2O/O_2.[65]
D. Patients undergoing prostate biopsy indicated that analgesia with Entonox provided effective analgesia.[66] The authors cited N_2O and O_2 as the analgesia of choice for this procedure.
E. Ujhelyi *et al* indicated no adverse events and full recovery when nitrous oxide was used with atrial defibrillation shocks.[67]

REFERENCES

1. Minnett RJ: Self-administered anaesthesia in childbirth, *BMJ* 1:501, 1934.
2. Baskett PJ, Withnell A: Use of Entonox on the ambulance service, *BMJ* 2:41, 1970.
3. Stewart RD: Nitrous oxide sedation/analgesia in emergency medicine, *Ann Emerg Med* 14:139, 1985.
4. Amey BD, Ballinger JA, Harrison EE: Prehospital administration of nitrous oxide for control of pain, *Ann Emerg Med* 10:247, 1981.
5. Pons PT: Nitrous oxide analgesia, *Emerg Med Clin North Am* 6:777, 1988.
6. Faddy SC, Garlick SR: A systematic review of the safety of analgesia with 50% nitrous oxide: can lay responders use analgesic gases in the prehospital setting? *Emerg Med J* 22:901, 2005.
7. Flomenbaum N *et al*: Self-administered nitrous oxide: an adjunct analgesic, *J Am Col Emerg Phys* 8:95, 1979.
8. Pinell MC, Linscott MS: Nitrous oxide in the emergency department, *Am J Emerg Med* 5:395, 1987.
9. Hayes GB: Relief of cardiac chest pain in the field, *Emerg Care Q* 3:49, 1987.
10. Gamis AS, Knapp JF, Glenski JA: Nitrous oxide analgesia in a pediatric emergency department, *Ann Emerg Med* 18:177, 1989.
11. Gerhardt RT *et al*: Inhaled nitrous oxide versus placebo as an analgesic and anxiolytic adjunct to peripheral intravenous cannulation, *Am J Emerg Med* 19(6):492, 2001.
12. Ekbom K, Jakobsson J, Marcus C: Nitrous oxide inhalation is a safe and effective way to facilitate procedures in paediatric outpatient departments, *Arch Dis Child* 90:1073, 2005.
13. White LJ *et al*: Prehospital use of analgesia for suspected extremity fractures, *Prehosp Emerg Care* 4(3):205, 2000.

14. Kennedy RM, Luhmann JD, Luhmann SJ: Emergency department management of pain and anxiety related to orthopedic fracture care: a guide to analgesic techniques and procedural sedation in children, *Pediatr Drugs* 6 (1):11, 2004.

15. Blasier RD: Anesthetic considerations for fracture management in the outpatient setting, *J Pediatr Orthop* 24 (6):742, 2004.

16. Marx GF, Katsnelson T: The introduction of nitrous oxide analgesia into obstetrics, *Obstet Gynecol* 80:715, 1992.

17. Santos AC, Pedersen H: Current controversies in obstetric anesthesia, *Anesth Anal* 78:753, 1994.

18. Arthurs GJ, Rosen M: Acceptability of continuous nasal nitrous oxide during labour: a field trial in six maternity hospitals, *Anaesthesia* 36:384, 1981.

19. Carstoniu J, Levytam S, Norman P: Nitrous oxide in early labor: safety and analgesic efficacy assessed by a double-blind, placebo-controlled study, *Anesthesiology* 80:30, 1994.

20. Fortescue C, Wee MYK: Analgesia in labour: non-regional techniques, *Cont Ed Anesth, Critical Care Pain* 5(1):9, 2005.

21. Vallejo MC *et al*: Nitrous oxide anxiolysis for elective cesarean section, *J Clin Anesth* 17:543, 2005.

22. Ohlgisser M, Sorokin Y, Heifetz M: Gynecologic laparoscopy, *Obstet Gynecol Surv* 40:385, 1985.

23. Sadick NS, Militana CJ: Use of nitrous oxide in hair transplantation surgery, *J Dermatol Surg Oncol* 20:186, 1994.

24. Boullie MC: Nitrous oxide cryosurgery applied to skin cancers, *Dermatol Surg* 23(8):714, 1997.

25. Klein JA: Anesthesia for liposuction in dermatologic surgery, *J Dermatol Surg Oncol* 14:1124, 1988.

26. Maloney JM, Coleman WP, Mora R: Analgesia induced by nitrous oxide and oxygen as an adjunct to local anesthesia in dermatologic surgery, *J Dermatol Surg Oncol* 6:939, 1980.

27. Arancia L: Nitrous oxide inhalation analgesia in ambulatory foot surgery, *J Am Coll Foot Surg* 5:111, 1966.

28. Mosher MR, Sorkin BS: Nitrous oxide/oxygen analgesia in podiatric surgery, *J Am Podiatry Assoc* 62:142, 1972.

29. Harris WC, Alpert WJ, Gill JJ: Nitrous oxide and Valium use in podiatric surgery for production of conscious-sedation, *J Am Podiatry Assoc* 72:505, 1982.

30. McMahan LB: Nitrous oxide analgesia for cataract surgery, *Ophthalmic Surg* 13:307, 1982.

31. Corboy JM: Nitrous oxide analgesia for outpatient surgery, *Am Intra-Ocular Implant Soc J* 10:232, 1984.

32. Thompson V: Personal communication, September 1997.

33. Sullivan JH: Cryosurgery in ophthalmic practice, *Ophthalmic Surg* 10:37, 1979.

34. Noppen M *et al*: Bronchoscopic cryotherapy: preliminary experience, *Acta Clinical Belg* 56(2):73, 2001.

35. Brill NW *et al*: Relative effectiveness of various forms of electroconvulsive therapy, *Arch Neurol Psychiatry* 81:109, 1959.

36. Gillman MA: Analgesic nitrous oxide as a therapeutic and investigative tool in neurological conditions. In Sinha KK, editor: *Progress in Clinical Neurosciences,* vol 2, Ranchi, 1985, Neurological Society of India.

37. Gillman MA, Lichtigfeld FJ: The effects of nitrous oxide and naloxone on orgasm in human females: a preliminary report, *J Sex Res* 19:49, 1986.

38. deWet J *et al*: Psychotropic analgesic nitrous oxide (PAN) for hyperactivity, *Aust N Z J Psychiatry* 35(4):543, 2001.

39. Diehl DL *et al*: Nitrous oxide (N_2O) vs intravenous sedation in upper gastrointestinal endoscopy (EGD): a prospective randomized controlled trial, *Gastrointest Endosc* 43:310, 1996.

40. Forbes GM, Collins BJ: Nitrous oxide for colonoscopy: a randomized controlled study, *Gastrointest Endosc* 51 (3):271, 2000.

41. Theodorou T *et al*: Total intravenous versus inhalational anaesthesia for colonoscopy: a prospective study of clinical recovery and psychomotor function, *Anaesth Intensive Care* 29:124, 2001.

42. Harding TA, Gibson JA: The use of inhaled nitrous oxide for flexible sigmoidoscopy: a placebo-controlled trial, *Endoscopy* 32:457, 2000.

43. Fauroux B *et al*: The efficacy of premixed nitrous oxide and oxygen for fiberoptic bronchoscopy in pediatric patients, *Chest* 125:315, 2004.

44. Kripke BJ, Hechtman HB: Nitrous oxide for pentazocine addiction and for intractable pain: report of case, *Anesth Analg* 51:520, 1972.

45. Lichtigfeld FJ, Gillman MA: The treatment of alcoholic withdrawal states with oxygen and nitrous oxide, *S Afr Med J* 61:349, 1982.

46. Gillman MA, Lichtigfeld FJ: Randomized double-blind trial of psychotropic analgesic nitrous oxide compared with diazepam for alcohol withdrawal state, *J Subst Abuse Treat* 22:129, 2002.

47. Gillman MA, Lichtigfeld FJ: Analgesic nitrous oxide in neuropsychiatry: past, present and future, *Intern J Neurosci* 49:75, 1989.
48. Katzen BT, Edwards KC: Nitrous-oxide analgesia for interventional radiologic procedures, *Am J Roentgenol* 140:145, 1983.
49. Ayer WA *et al*: Overcoming dental fear: strategies for its prevention and management, *JADA* 107:18, 1983.
50. Malamed SF: Sedation, *A Guide to Patient Management*, ed 4, St. Louis, 2003, Mosby.
51. Chidiac JJ *et al*: Gagging prevention using nitrous oxide or table salt: a comparative pilot study, *Int J Prosth* 14 (4):364, 2001.
52. Packer ME, Joarder C, Lall BA: The use of relative analgesia in the prosthetic treatment of the "gagging" patient, *Dent Update* 32:544, 2005.
53. Davis MJ: Conscious sedation practices in pediatric dentistry: a survey of members of the American Board of Pediatric Dentistry College of Diplomates, *Pediatr Dent* 10:328, 1988.
54. Griffin GC, Campbell VD, Jones R: Nitrous oxide-oxygen sedation for minor surgery, *JAMA* 245:2411, 1981.
55. Iosava KV: Analgesic anesthesia with nitrous oxide in pain syndrome caused by coronary insufficiency (clinico-biochemical studies), *Kardiologiia* 5:54, 1965.
56. Pekker IL: Nitrous oxide anesthesia with pipolphan pre-medication in myocardial infarct at a first aid station, *Sov Med* 28:103, 1965.
57. Keer F *et al*: Nitrous oxide analgesia in myocardial infarction, *Lancet* 1:63, 1972.
58. Thompson PL, Lown B: Nitrous oxide as an analgesic in acute myocardial infarction, *JAMA* 235:924, 1976.
59. Iannalfi A *et al*: Painful procedures in children with cancer: comparison of moderate sedation and general anesthesia for lumbar puncture and bone marrow aspiration, *Pediatr Blood Cancer* 45:933, 2005.
60. Foley KM: The treatment of pain in the patient with cancer, *CA Cancer J Clin* 36:194, 1986.
61. Fosburg MT, Crone RK: Nitrous oxide analgesia for refractory pain in the terminally ill, *JAMA* 250:511, 1983.
62. Keating HJ III, Kundrat M: Patient-controlled analgesia with nitrous oxide in cancer pain, *J Pain Symptom Manage* 11:126, 1996.
63. Castera L *et al*: Patient-administered nitrous oxide/oxygen inhalation provides safe and effective analgesia for percutaneous liver biopsy: a randomized placebo-controlled trial, *Am J Gastroenterology* 96(5):1553, 2001.
64. Stanley A: Migraine treated by inhalation sedation using nitrous oxide and oxygen, *Brit Dent J* 149:54, 1980.
65. Triner WR *et al*: Nitrous oxide for the treatment of acute migraine headache, *Am J Emerg Med* 17(3):252, 1999.
66. Masood J *et al*: Nitrous oxide (Entonox) inhalation and tolerance of transrectal ultrasound guided prostate biopsy: a double-blind randomized controlled study, *J Urology* 168:116, 2002.
67. Ujhelyi M *et al*: Nitrous oxide sedation reduces discomfort caused by atrial defibrillation shocks, *PACE* 27:485, 2004.

SUGGESTED READINGS

Cruickshank JC, Sykes SH: Office sedation, *Adv Dermatol* 7:291, 1992.
Edwards FJ: The art of sedation in the emergency department, *J Am Acad Phys Assist* 7:128, 1994.
Henderson JM *et al*: Administration of nitrous oxide to pediatric patients provides analgesia for venous cannulation, *Anesthesiology* 72:269, 1990.
Hovorka J, Korttila K: Nitrous oxide does not increase nausea and vomiting following gynaecological laparoscopy, *Can J Anaesth* 36:145, 1989.
Miller K: Analgesia: issues and options, *Emergency* 21:16, 1989.
Thal ER *et al*: Self-administered analgesia with nitrous oxide: adjunctive aid for emergency medical care systems, *JAMA* 242:2418, 1979.
Toulson S: More than a lot of hot air, *Nursing* 4:23, 1990.
Tunstall ME: Implications of pre-mixed gases and apparatus for their administration, *Br J Anaesth* 40:675, 1968.
Werty EM: Pediatric conscious sedation, *Emergency* 25:19, 1994.

Chapter 16

Clinical Application of N_2O/O_2 Sedation in Pediatrics

Young children live in a magical world. The thoughts and activities in their world are experienced with an unprejudiced mind and heart. Unfortunately, adults often inadvertently transfer negative attitudes of medical/dental procedures to children. N_2O/O_2 sedation produces a unique euphoria that provides and reinforces a positive attitude toward healthcare in the pediatric patient. Recent evidence suggests that most pediatric dentists routinely use N_2O/O_2 sedation in their practices.[1] Thus, it can only be concluded that it is great for kids.

I. CHILD DEVELOPMENT

A. Piaget proposed a model for child development that addresses cognitive function or how a child thinks. According to Piaget, children move through four stages of development: sensorimotor, preoperational, concrete operational, and formal operational. He proposed that for cognitive development, the movement from stage to stage is universal and invariant (proceeding in a fixed order)[2] (Table 16-1).

B. These stages give clues about how children should be approached if they are developing normally. Similar to adults, it is common for pediatric patients to have some anxiety regarding medical or dental treatment.

C. There are additional significant factors that affect the development of a child today. Changing patterns of child rearing, parental interactions and attitudes toward professionals, and individual child temperament and personality affect the way a child acts and reacts in any given setting.

D. It is important for health professionals and office staff to be educated about these factors, because understanding the pediatric patient's needs and desires and those of the parents is imperative.

II. AAP/AAPD JOINT GUIDELINES[3]

The American Academy of Pediatrics (AAP) and the American Academy of Pediatric Dentistry (AAPD) have jointly published guidelines intended for those practitioners who deliver sedation to children. These guidelines were developed in response to the increase in invasive diagnostic and minor surgical procedures being completed either on an elective or emergency basis in settings outside of the operating room. These guidelines provide a unified stance regarding sedation for both medical and dental practitioners.[3] This current statement underscores the need for careful preprocedural evaluation, appropriate fasting, airway evaluation, and appropriately trained individuals capable of monitoring the patient, as well as knowledge of associated risks, because sedation is different for children than adults. The document also reinforces safety as a primary concern and emphasizes the fact that the ability to rescue a child from the deeper level than that intended is imperative.[3]

Table 16-1. Piaget's Stages of Child Development

Phase	Language	Fears	Defenses
Sensorimotor Under 18 months	Minimal	Sudden noises New situations Separation from parents	Cry, scream Move away
Preoperational 2–4 years	Developing vocabulary, grammar, language	Not well understood Monsters Dark	Magical Not rational
Preoperational 5–6 years	Language better Simple vocabulary	Can react with shame	Moves away from situation, denial
Operational 7–12 years	Excellent in concrete understanding Abstract less developed	Fears more realistic Fears loss of control Fear of death	Restrained; developing internal defenses
Formal 12–18 years	Full development with language	Mirror adult world Fear of getting hurt Fears of world affairs	Intellectual and rational

A. **Terminology**
1. The American Society of Anesthesiologists, the Joint Commission on Accreditation of Healthcare Organizations, the AAP, and the AAPD all use similar language with regard to the definitions of sedation categories.
2. The definitions of minimal, moderate, deep, and general anesthesia can be found in Chapter 3.

B. **Goals of sedation**
1. The goals of sedation as listed in this document include (1) guarding the patient's safety and welfare, (2) minimizing physical discomfort and pain, (3) controlling anxiety and maximizing amnestic potential, (4) controlling behavior and movement, and (5) returning the patient to a state where discharge is safe.[3]
2. Selecting the lowest dose of drug, the fewest number of drugs, and the correct drug to meet the intended goal of accomplishing the procedure is recommended.[3]

C. **General guidelines[3]**
1. The AAP/AAPD recommend sedating children who fall in the ASA classes of I and II. Those individuals in the III and IV classes or who have special needs or abnormal airways should be carefully considered.
2. A responsible adult should accompany a child to and from an appointment, and care should be taken to ensure adequate monitoring of those who would need to travel in a car seat. Caution for this situation corresponds to the potential for a child's head to fall forward and obstruct the airway.
3. These recommendations indicate that the facilities and personnel should be able to manage all emergency and rescue situations. Appropriate training is necessary, and emergency equipment must be available at the facility and able to be appropriately used if needed.
4. Informed consent from the responsible accompanying adult must be obtained before any procedure. In addition, all instructions regarding the procedure should be complete while giving the adult ample opportunity to ask questions.

5. If immobilization devices are used, they are to be carefully positioned so that airway obstruction or chest restriction is avoided.

III. N_2O/O_2 USE IN PEDIATRICS

A. Pediatric dentistry

1. The specialty of pediatric dentistry was established in 1948. The reason was simple and quite clear. Children are not small adults in anatomy, physiology, or behavior, and they require separate consideration for evaluation, management, and treatment.

2. Wilson[1] reported in a 1993 survey of the membership of the AAPD that 89% of the 1758 respondents used N_2O to treat pediatric patients.

  a. Of those who used N_2O/O_2, most practitioners (87%) used the titration method of administration.

  b. The percentage of N_2O administered varied; however, rarely did concentrations exceed 50%.[1]

  c. Most respondents indicated that 20% or fewer of their patients required either N_2O/O_2 alone or in combination with other sedatives.[1]

  d. Wilson reported that 74% of the respondents did not use any monitors when N_2O/O_2 was used alone. However, when it was used in combination with other sedatives, the pulse oximeter was the single most frequently used monitoring device. A blood pressure cuff and stethoscope were also used when N_2O was combined with other sedatives.[1]

  e. When N_2O/O_2 was used alone, only 2% of the respondents had ever experienced a compromised airway. When deeper sedation was achieved by use of N_2O with other sedatives, the figure affirming experience with a compromised airway rose only to one third.[1]

3. Houpt has also surveyed the membership of the AAPD over the years as to the use of sedative agents by pediatric dentists.[4] Wide variation among practitioners exists as to the use of sedation agents and their frequency. The figures in this 15-year follow-up survey reflect that N_2O is still used by practitioners and use has increased in those who use sedation frequently.[4]

4. N_2O/O_2 significantly modifies uncooperative behaviors[5,6] but not physiologic parameters in sedated children.[7,8]

5. Internationally, N_2O and O_2 are being used successfully.[9–11] Foley indicated that the extraction of first permanent molars can be accomplished successfully with N_2O/O_2 sedation.[12] It has also been advocated as a potential alternative to general anesthesia when treating children.[13–15]

6. Primosch *et al* demonstrated that the delivery of a 40% N_2O/60% O_2 combination significantly improved patient behavior without significantly affecting hemoglobin saturation or type of breath sound.[16]

7. N_2O has been used concomitantly with other drugs, such as sevoflurane and midazolam.[17–20] Although success and effectiveness were demonstrated, Cote reported that adverse sedation events were associated with drug overdoses and interactions when combinations of drugs were administered.[21]

B. Emergency medicine

1. The use of N_2O in the emergency department has been evaluated for children undergoing procedures such as fracture management, laceration repair, intravenous cannulation, and other minor surgical procedures.[22–25]

2. Researchers acknowledge the anxiety associated with these procedures and the possibility of N_2O to be an effective, noninvasive way to reduce anxiety with minimal adverse effects.[22,26,27]

3. In cases in which N_2O/O_2 alone was used during fracture reduction, the procedure was successful, but children reported pain.[28] Hennrikus[28] reported greater success when he combined N_2O with a hematoma block to provide additional analgesia.
4. During laceration repair, continuous-flow N_2O/O_2 provided pain and anxiety relief with minimal adverse effects and shorter recovery than when midazolam was used.[29]

C. **Endoscopy**
1. The use of N_2O/O_2 for pediatric patients undergoing gastrointestinal endoscopy has been evaluated in a pilot study in France. Investigators noted the rapid and effective analgesia without heavy sedation in addition to a short recovery period.[30]
2. Fauroux also evaluated the efficacy of N_2O and O_2 compared with nitrogen and O_2 during fiberoptic bronchoscopy procedures in pediatric patients.[31] Researchers noted better sedation and pain control with N_2O and O_2.
3. It is important to keep in mind that the use of 50% N_2O and 50% O_2 as a standard method of administration is contrary to the best and most effective administration technique.

D. **Painful procedures**
1. N_2O/O_2 has proven beneficial for pediatric patients who must undergo repeated painful procedures, such as venous cannulation, bone marrow aspiration, lumbar punctures, and dressing changes.[32,33]
2. The most favorable characteristics cited were short recovery time and amnestic effects.

E. **Otologic examination**
1. Suctioning ears and other otomicroscopic examining procedures prove to be uncomfortable for children. Fishman cited success in 21 of 24 patients treated with N_2O and O_2.[34]
2. In addition, researchers also indicated there was no need for physical restraint with this type of sedation.

IV. PEDIATRIC PATIENT CONSIDERATIONS FOR USE OF N_2O/O_2 SEDATION

A. The attitude of the practitioner and staff is the single most important factor in the successful administration of N_2O/O_2 to pediatric patients.
B. Spontaneous cooperation and willingness of the patient to accept treatment is clearly one of the most important factors to consider.
C. Equally as important is whether the patient can and will respond to reason.
D. It must be determined whether the intended treatment can be accomplished with N_2O/O_2 sedation or whether additional pharmacologic management is required.
E. N_2O/O_2 sedation does not require an extensive physical evaluation of the child; however, the AAP/AAPD recommends a comprehensive health evaluation.[3]
1. The health evaluation should include a history of allergies, medication or drugs taken, diseases and abnormalities, pregnancy status, hospitalizations, previous sedation experiences, and other relevant information related to anesthesia.[3]
2. Anatomic factors that affect the respiratory system, such as enlarged tonsils and adenoids, are of relative importance because they can cause increased resistance to gas movement.
3. In children, middle ear disturbances can become an important factor to consider because N_2O can aggravate these conditions.[35]
4. Advise parents to have children avoid eating a heavy meal before the appointment, because sedatives have the potential to affect protective airway reflexes.
   a. Pediatric patients are far more likely to regurgitate than adults.
   b. Aspiration of vomitus is rare but is a very serious and potentially fatal situation.

     c. Let patients vomit if they need to vomit. If vomiting occurs, the mouth must be suctioned and the child's airway cleared of vomitus.

     d. Fasting guidelines can be found in Chapter 10.

F. Weight is usually a most important factor in the administration of proper medication dosages for patients, particularly children. However, weight is not a consideration for N_2O/O_2 administration.

V. ADMINISTRATION OF N_2O/O_2 SEDATION TO PEDIATRIC PATIENTS

A. The AAP/AAPD guidelines recommend the use of a systematic approach before sedation. The acronym "SOAPME" offers a routine for preparing for sedation. See Box 16-1. The acronym stands for suction, oxygen, airway, pharmacy, monitors, and equipment.[3]

B. The specific technique of administration does not differ from that of the adult. In 2005, the AAPD published the "Guideline on Appropriate Use of Nitrous Oxide for Pediatric Dental Patients."[36]

    1. N_2O/O_2 must be administered only by appropriately licensed individuals.

    2. Informed consent must be obtained from the parent and documented in the patient's record before administration of N_2O/O_2.

    3. Preoperative and postoperative vital sign values are to be recorded.

    4. Select the nasal hood according to the size of the individual. All child patients should be encouraged to touch, examine, and place the nasal hood on the nose before N_2O administration. Make sure it fits snugly. This can decrease patient anxiety and increase trust in the practitioner (Figures 16-1 and 16-2). Items to distract the child's attention are always beneficial (Figure 16-3).

    5. Determine the flow rate for each person. Typically, a rate of 5–6 L/min is acceptable for most patients. Establish the flow rate by observing the reservoir bag while delivering 100% O_2. The bag should pulsate gently with inspiration and exhalation and should not be either overinflated or underinflated. Reservoir bags are available in smaller sizes (e.g., 1–2 L) that accommodate tidal volumes of pediatric patients.

    6. Titration is the single most important concept to follow. Titration of N_2O in 10% intervals is recommended.[36] Like adults, children will exhibit signs and symptoms of sedation (Figure 16-4). It is important to remember to allow time between the increments so the drug can reach its peak effect before adding more; this will avoid oversedation.

Box 16-1	**PREPARATION FOR SEDATION PROCEDURES**

S (suction)—size-appropriate suction catheters and a functioning suction apparatus (e.g., Yankauer-type suction).

O (oxygen)—adequate oxygen supply and functioning flowmeters/other devices to allow its delivery.

A (airway)—size-appropriate airway equipment (nasopharyngeal and oropharyngeal airways, laryngoscope blades [checked and functioning], endotracheal tubes, stylets, face mask, bag-valve-mask or equivalent device).

P (pharmacy)—all the basic drugs needed to support life during an emergency, including antagonists as indicated.

M (monitors)—functioning pulse oximeter with size-appropriate oximeter probes and other monitors as appropriate for the procedure (e.g., noninvasive blood pressure, end-tidal carbon dioxide, ECG, stethoscope).

E (equipment)—special equipment or drugs for a particular case (e.g., defibrillator).

From the American Academy of Pediatrics and the American Academy of Pediatric Dentistry Guidelines for Monitoring and Management of Pediatric Patients During and After Sedation for Diagnostic and Therapeutic Procedures: An Update, Dec. 2006.

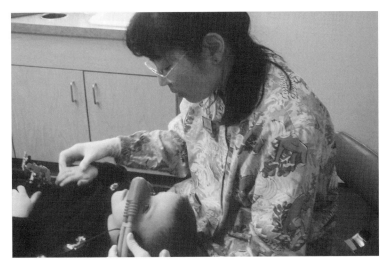

Figure 16-1 Place the nasal hood on the child and encourage him or her to become acquainted with the hood. *(Photo by Dr. Morris Clark.)*

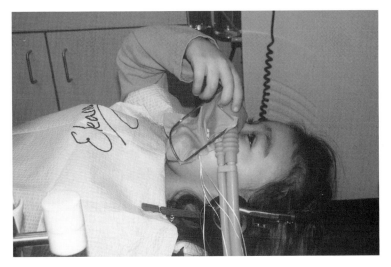

Figure 16-2 Allow the child to touch the nasal hood and adjust it if necessary. *(Photo by Dr. Morris Clark.)*

7. It is typically not necessary for the concentration of N_2O to exceed 50%. The concentration of nitrous oxide may be decreased or increased depending on the intensity of the procedure. Avoid the "roller coaster" effect of sharp increases and decreases in concentrations of N_2O administered. This can make the patient feel nauseous or feel unpleasant about the entire experience. If patients become nauseous, turn down the N_2O and increase the O_2 flow.

8. During treatment, it is important to continue the visual monitoring of the patient's respiratory rate and level of consciousness.[36]

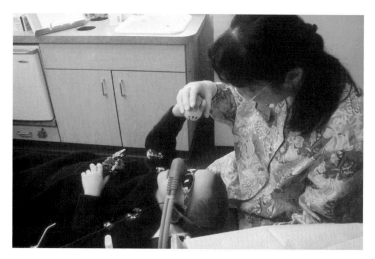

Figure 16-3 Distraction diverts attention. *(Photo by Dr. Morris Clark.)*

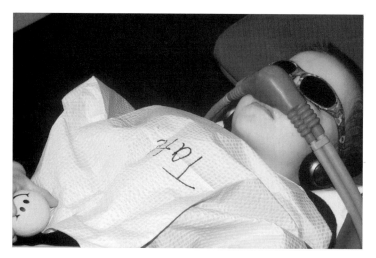

Figure 16-4 Child is relaxed and comfortable. *(Photo by Dr. Morris Clark.)*

9. Pulse oximetry is commonly used today, and the equipment is relatively inexpensive. A pulse oximeter is not mandatory for N_2O/O_2 sedation. It may be used as an additional means to monitor a patient when high concentrations of N_2O are used.[36]

10. Once the nitrous oxide flow is terminated, 100% O_2 should be delivered for a minimum of 5 minutes. Appropriate recovery must be demonstrated, and the patient must return to pretreatment responsiveness before he or she is dismissed.

C. The rapid induction technique method of administration has been advocated to gain the attention and cooperation or regain the composure of young children.

1. High concentrations of N_2O (50% or greater) are administered to children, typically ages 3 years and younger.

2. With this technique, crying can be minimized, initially and temporarily. This "settling" phase is short-lived in most cases and allows the child to regain composure.
3. After composure has been attained, the concentration should be reduced.
4. "Crashing" or giving high concentrations of N_2O initially until an injection is given is a technique used by many pediatric dentists with success in very young children.
    a. Remember that N_2O has its own analgesic effects.
    b. This fact should be recognized and used during the injection phase of treatment.
    c. Although local anesthetics have sedative properties, they are not considered sedatives and can be combined with nitrous oxide/oxygen (Figure 16-5). However, if other sedating medications are used, such as chloral hydrate, midazolam, or an opioid, the likelihood for the child to enter moderate or deep sedation is greater.[36]

D. Houpt *et al* observed the clinical effects of nitrous oxide in children.[37] Most children (70%) reported feeling good, and a variety of sensations were described. Several children reported sensations in their extremities, abdomen, and lips. Some reported warmth, lightness, or heaviness.[37] It was observed that children had open hands (90%) and limp legs (81%).[37] Children were also observed smiling with a trancelike expression; laughter occurred in some (Figure 16-6).[37]
E. Positive reinforcement (e.g., material or social reward) is usually given for participating rather than how the child participated during a routine visit to a medical or dental office.
F. Recovery must be complete before a child can be dismissed (Figure 16-7). The AAPD recommends the following criteria be observed before discharge:
    1. Vital signs are within normal range and parallel values obtained preoperatively to ensure stable physiology.
    2. Airway is patent and uncompromised.
    3. Patient is easily aroused with intact protective gag and cough reflexes.
    4. Patient can talk, sit up, and walk without assistance, if applicable.

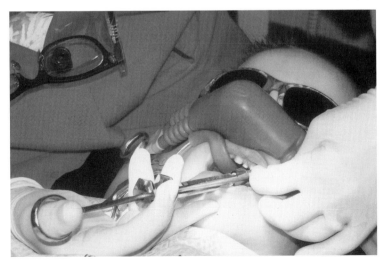

Figure 16-5 Local anesthesia combined with N_2O/O_2.

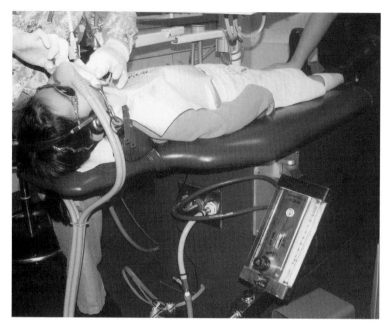

Figure 16-6 Appropriate pediatric sedation with N_2O/O_2.

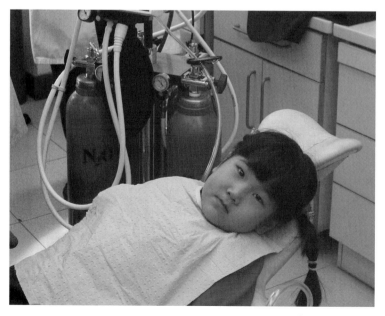

Figure 16-7 Recovery is complete. *(Courtesy Dr. Jack Chen and Dr. Zheng Wei.)*

5. The postsedation level of responsiveness closely parallels that of presedation.
6. Child is discharged to an appropriate, responsible individual.[38]

G. Documentation is mandatory for all pediatric sedation procedures just as it is for adults. All aspects of the sedation record must be completed similarly whether treating a child or adult. See an example of a sedation record in Appendix C.

VI. SAFETY OF PEDIATRIC PATIENTS

A. All patients are important, and their safety and welfare are the first priority. However, it is the pediatric patient who captures all of the practitioner's senses of concern and responsibility. An emergency is especially emotionally charged when a child is involved. N$_2$O/O$_2$ provides a measure of safety that practitioners seek when treating pediatric patients.

B. It is not advised to let the child fall asleep under N$_2$O/O$_2$ sedation.
1. Silent regurgitation is the most engaging concern in this situation.
2. Maintaining conversation with the child ensures the protective laryngeal and pharyngeal reflexes are intact and the child is able to cough.
3. If a child does fall asleep, a pretracheal scope will alert the practitioner that the airway is not patent.

C. Parents are generally dismissed before the procedure starts if the child is 3 years old or older.
1. Separation breaks the dependent psychologic bond that can worsen a fearful situation. Parents who insist on staying in the operatory are requested to be passive observers.
2. Parents must be informed in detail about the procedure and that the child should be 100% recovered and alert on discharge.
3. Informed consent must be obtained from the parents for each N$_2$O/O$_2$ administration. Tahir reported a significant observation regarding parental consent. It was discovered that 40% of consent obtained was not valid, because the parents did not fully understand what they were consenting to even after a full explanation of the treatment and type of anesthesia their child was to undergo.[39]

D. Concomitant use of other agents with N$_2$O is a matter of practitioner choice. However, it is important to know the pharmacology of the drugs used and their interaction with each other.

VII. APPOINTMENT LENGTH

A. Depending on his or her age, personality, and/or systematic health, a child's attention span is minimal and can rarely be maintained beyond 45 minutes.

B. Do not prolong pediatric appointments. It is important to remember not to prolong appointments with children whether N$_2$O/O$_2$ sedation is being used or not.

REFERENCES

1. Wilson S: A survey of the American Academy of Pediatric Dentistry membership: nitrous oxide and sedation, *Pediatr Dent* 18:287, 1995.
2. Piaget J, Inhelder B: *The Psychology of the Child*, New York, 1969, Basic Books.
3. Cote CJ, Wilson S: American Academy of Pediatrics and American Academy of Pediatric Dentistry: Guidelines for monitoring and management of pediatric patients during and after sedation for diagnostic and therapeutic procedures: an update, *Pediatrics* 118(6):2587, 2006.
4. Houpt M: Project USAP 2000—Use of sedative agents by pediatric dentists: a 15-year follow-up survey, *Ped Dent* 24(4):289, 2002.

5. Foley J: Nitrous oxide inhalation sedation: what do patients, carers and dentists think about it? *Eur J Paediatr Dent* 6(1):23, 2005.
6. Collado V *et al*: Modification of behavior with 50% nitrous oxide/oxygen conscious sedation over repeated visits for dental treatment: a 3-year prospective study, *J Clin Psychopharm* 26(5):474, 2006.
7. Wilson S *et al*: The effects of nitrous oxide on pediatric dental patients sedated with chloral hydrate and hydroxyzine, *Ped Dent* 20(4):253, 1998.
8. Leelataweewud P *et al*: The physiological effects of supplemental oxygen versus nitrous oxide/oxygen during conscious sedation of pediatric dental patients, *Ped Dent* 22(2):125, 2000.
9. Peretz B: The use of sedation while treating paediatric dental patients in Israel, *Int J Paed Dent* 12:355, 2002.
10. Klinkberg G: Pharmacological approach to the management of dental anxiety in children—comments from a Scandinavian point of view, *Int J Paed Dent* 12:357, 2002.
11. Folayan MO *et al*: A review of the pharmacological approach to the management of dental anxiety in children, *Int J Paed Dent* 12:347, 2002.
12. Foley J: Efficacy of nitrous oxide inhalation sedation and first permanent molar tooth extractions, *SAAD* 23:3, 2007.
13. Paterson SA, Tahmassebi JF: Pediatric dentistry in the new millennium: 3. Use of inhalation sedation in paediatric dentistry, *Dent Update* 30(7):350, 2003.
14. Hosey MT: Managing anxious children: the use of conscious sedation in paediatric dentistry, *Int J Paed Dent* 12:359, 2002.
15. Lyratzopoulos G, Blain KM: Inhalation sedation with nitrous oxide as an alternative to dental general anaesthesia for children, *J Pub Health Med* 25(4):303, 2003.
16. Primosch RE *et al*: Effect of nitrous oxide-oxygen inhalation with scavenging on behavioral and physiological parameters during routine dental treatment, *Pediatr Dent* 21(7):417, 1999.
17. Hulland SA *et al*: Nitrous oxide-oxygen or oral midazolam for pediatric outpatient sedation, *Oral Surg Oral Med Oral Pathol Oral Radiol Endod* 93:643, 2002.
18. Averley PA *et al*: A randomised controlled trial of paediatric conscious sedation for dental treatment using intravenous midazolam combined with inhaled nitrous oxide or nitrous oxide/sevoflurane, *Anaesthesia* 59:844, 2004.
19. Lahoud GY, Averley PA: Comparison of sevoflurane and nitrous oxide mixture with nitrous oxide alone for inhalation conscious sedation in children having dental treatment: a randomised controlled trial, *Anaesthesia* 57:446, 2002.
20. Otley CC, Nguyen TH: Conscious sedation of pediatric patients with combination oral benzodiazepines and inhaled nitrous oxide, *Dermatol Surg* 26(11):1041, 2000.
21. Cote CJ *et al*: Adverse sedation events in pediatrics: analysis of medications used for sedation, *Pediatrics* 106 (4):633, 2000.
22. Krauss B: Continuous-flow nitrous oxide: searching for the ideal procedural anxiolytic for toddlers, *Ann Emerg Med* 37(1):61, 2001.
23. Griffin G *et al*: Nitrous oxide-oxygen sedation for minor surgery: experience in a pediatric setting, *JAMA* 245:2411, 1983.
24. Gamis AS *et al*: Nitrous oxide analgesia in a pediatric emergency department, *Ann Emerg Med* 18:177, 1989.
25. Kennedy RM, Luhmann JD: Pharmacological management of pain and anxiety during emergency procedures in children, *Paediatr Drugs* 3(5):337, 2001.
26. Frampton A *et al*: Nurse administered relative analgesia using high concentration nitrous oxide to facilitate minor procedures in children in an emergency department, *Emerg Med J* 20:410, 2003.
27. Burnweit C *et al*: Nitrous oxide analgesia for minor pediatric surgical procedures: an effective alternative to conscious sedation? *J Ped Surg* 39(3):495, 2004.
28. Hennrikus WL: Self-administered nitrous oxide analgesia for pediatric fracture reductions, *J Pediatr Orthop* 14:538, 1994.
29. Luhmann JD *et al*: A randomized clinical trial of continuous-flow nitrous oxide and midazolam for sedation of young children during laceration repair, *Ann Emerg Med* 37(1):20, 2001.
30. Michaud L: Nitrous oxide sedation in pediatric patients undergoing gastrointestinal endoscopy, *J Pediatr Gastroenterol Nutr.* 28(3):310, 1999.
31. Fauroux B *et al*: The efficacy of premixed nitrous oxide and oxygen for fiberoptic bronchoscopy in pediatric patients, *Chest* 125(1):315, 2004.
32. Kanagasundaram SA *et al*: Efficacy and safety of nitrous oxide in alleviating pain and anxiety during painful procedures, *Arch Dis Child* 84(6):492, 2001.

33. O'Brian L *et al:* Pharmacologic management of painful oncology procedures in pediatrics, *Am J Cancer* 2 (6):403, 2003.
34. Fishman G *et al:* Nitrous oxide-oxygen inhalation for outpatient otologic examination and minor procedures performed on the uncooperative child, *Int J Ped Otorhinolaryng* 69:501, 2005.
35. Munson ES: Complications of nitrous oxide anesthesia for ear surgery, *Anes Clin North Am* 11(3):559, 1993.
36. American Academy of Pediatric Dentistry Council on Clinical Affairs: Guideline on appropriate use of nitrous oxide for pediatric dental patients, *Ped Dent* 27:107, 2005.
37. Houpt MI *et al:* Clinical effects of nitrous oxide conscious sedation in children, *Ped Dent* 26(1):29, 2004.
38. American Academy of Pediatric Dentistry Committee on Sedation and Anesthesia: *Guideline on the Elective Use of Minimal, Moderate, and Deep Sedation and General Anesthesia for Pediatric Dental Patients,* Chicago, 2004, American Academy of Pediatric Dentistry.
39. Tahir MA *et al:* Informed consent: optimism versus reality, *Brit Dent J* 193(4):221, 2002.

Part III

ISSUES OF SPECIAL CONSIDERATION

Potential Biohazards for Health Personnel Associated with Chronic Exposure to N_2O

N_2O/O_2 sedation has already been discussed as a safe procedure that does not pose health risks for patients. However, chronic exposure for health professionals administering the gas has been an issue of debate and concern. This chapter provides current and accurate information to clarify this sometimes misunderstood and emotional issue.

I. HISTORY OF CONTROVERSIAL LITERATURE

A. In 1967, a scientist named Vaisman[1] reported that both male and female anesthesiologists in Russia experienced reproductive problems at a significantly higher rate than the general population. In addition, Vaisman concluded that these problems were caused by the occupational hazard of being chronically exposed to anesthetic gases. Because N_2O was a common denominator in most anesthetic applications, it was implicated as the causative agent.

B. In the United States, Cohen et al[2-4] published articles in the 1970s dealing with anesthetic health hazards. One 1980 published study[5] surveyed more than 50,000 dentists and dental assistants who were exposed to trace anesthetics. The results suggested that long-term exposure to anesthetic gases could be associated with an increase in general health problems and reproductive difficulty. In this study, ambient N_2O in the office was not measured, and data were collected through memory recall by dental personnel.

C. Since Vaisman's original article, the literature has continued to document and describe potential adverse effects of chronic exposure to N_2O. However, this literature has been primarily retrospective; therefore, inherent biases in study design were inevitable.[6] Because of these flaws, a definitive relationship between the exposure of an individual to N_2O/O_2 and reproductive sequelae cannot be established. Weinberg et al[7] addressed these design flaws and proposed recommendations for future studies of this sort.

D. Also during the 1970s, Bruce et al[8] investigated the possibility of N_2O affecting perceptual cognition and psychomotor skills of personnel exposed to varying concentrations of the gas. Their results were widely noted, because they reported audiovisual impairment in just hours of exposure to as little as 50 parts per million (ppm). Multiple attempts to reproduce the research results of Bruce et al have failed; interestingly, these researchers have retracted their conclusions, indicating the results were not based on biologic factors.[9] The National Institute for Occupational Safety and Health (NIOSH) became interested in these and other results being published and in 1977 evaluated the scavenging potential of the equipment used in both the operating room and the outpatient setting. It was determined that 25 ppm was achievable in the operating room but not attainable in a setting such as a dental operatory. Therefore, NIOSH chose 50 ppm to be the maximum exposure limit for personnel in a dental setting.[10] Although this limit has not been strictly enforced by the Occupational Safety and Health Administration (OSHA), it remains the recommended standard to date.

E. Despite the negative publicity N_2O received, other studies in the literature claimed no deleterious health effects associated with chronic exposure to N_2O, especially in low concentrations.[11-13] The controversy continued in the literature and was the subject at professional meetings. Both sides of the issue were published; however, because the effects were questionable, the popularity of N_2O/O_2 sedation waned.

F. It became the work of this author to objectively and scientifically evaluate all the published research to verify the possible relationship of chronic exposure to N_2O and its subsequent effects on human health.

   1. In 1995, a worldwide literature search on the topic of biohazards associated with N_2O use was conducted at the University of Colorado. Eight hundred fifty citations were retrieved, of which 23 met the predetermined criteria for scientific merit.

   2. The conclusions drawn from this literature review clearly indicated that there was no scientific basis for the previously established threshold levels for the hospital operating room or the dental setting.

   3. This research became the basis for a meeting of interested parties representing dentistry, government, and manufacturing. A result of the September 1995 meeting, which was sponsored by the ADA's Council on Scientific Affairs and Council on Dental Practice, was the formal position statement that a maximum N_2O exposure limit in parts per million has not been determined.[14] A subsequent report from this meeting indicates that the ADA urges governmental agencies to create new recommendations or regulations dealing with N_2O exposure that are science based.

II. SPECIFIC BIOLOGIC ISSUES AND HEALTH CONCERNS

A. Inactivation of methionine synthase is mentioned in Chapters 9, 17, and 18. N_2O interferes with this enzyme, which is linked to vitamin B_{12} metabolism. Vitamin B_{12} is necessary for DNA production and subsequent cellular reproduction.

   1. Inactivation of methionine synthase occurs rapidly in rats; exposure to 80% N_2O for only 15 minutes revealed inactivation of the enzyme.[15] Because of this interference, it was postulated that fetal development might be impaired because of exposure to N_2O. Animal studies that used approximately 60% N_2O for 24 hours on pregnant rats produced miscarriage and other fetal abnormalities.[16]

   2. Despite flawed research designs, there has been evidence that chronic exposure to high levels of N_2O does have an effect on reproduction.[5] However, to date no evidence that a direct causal relationship exists between reproductive health and scavenged low levels of N_2O has been found.[13,15]

   3. The deoxyuridine suppression test is a sensitive test used to accurately determine the first signs of biologic effect associated with chronic exposure to N_2O. The test detects the early signs of inactivation of the enzyme methionine synthase. By use of this test, Nunn *et al*[17] found that no alteration of this enzyme occurred in anesthetists exposed to between 150 and 400 ppm.

   4. In their research, Sweeney *et al*[18] showed that the first sign of biologic effect with the deoxyuridine suppression test was at a chronic exposure level of 1800 ppm. Experts in the field concur that the level of 400 ppm, suggested by Sweeney *et al*, is a reasonable exposure level that is both attainable and significantly below the biologic threshold established by Sweeney *et al*. The Health and Safety Executive in the United Kingdom (HSE UK) Occupation Exposure Limits set a figure of 100 ppm as a time-weighted average for 8 hours.[19] Other countries' exposure limits range from 25 ppm in France and Denmark to 100 ppm in Sweden and Germany.

5. Because of the significant demands for folic acid during organogenesis (first trimester), postponement of N_2O sedation is recommended. For a pregnant female employed in a setting that uses N_2O, it is important to know the exposure levels of N_2O and to use all recommended trace gas scavenging methods. Depending on the individual and the situation, that employee should determine whether she should avoid the office setting and any N_2O exposure for the first trimester.

B. Megaloblastic anemia, first described in the 1950s, was found in patients treated with N_2O for tetanus.[20] Leukopenia and reduced megaloblastic erythropoiesis resembling pernicious anemia ensued. Discussions continue as to the toxicity of nitrous oxide and its effects on the body.[21–28] It continues to seem that nitrous oxide is safe when administered in low therapeutic doses for short periods of time.

C. Neurologic disorders associated with chronic N_2O exposure appear as myeloneuropathy. Symptoms such as sensory and proprioception impairment may be permanent but are usually temporary with slow recovery.

III. LITERATURE REVIEW

A. Articles published in the 1990s refer primarily to scavenged versus unscavenged N_2O levels. In the 1990s, practitioners were educated on ways to effectively scavenge trace gas contamination, with the primary method being the evacuation system and the scavenging nasal hood or mask.

    1. The scavenging mask system has become standard on all product lines in the United States. When expired N_2O is exhaled through the nose, vacuum suction ports transport this gas through the central suction to the outside atmosphere (Figure 17-1). Studies evaluating the scavenging efficacy of masks indicate that current models significantly reduce the amount of trace N_2O in the ambient air.[29,30]

    2. This evacuation flow rate has been established by NIOSH as optimal at 45 L/min.

    3. Improved mask designs and/or evacuation devices are being investigated as modifications or additions to the current market.[31–35] As technology advances rapidly, no doubt there will be more efficient products. Ongoing research in this area is encouraged.

B. The published literature has served as a vehicle for informing healthcare professionals of the necessity to analyze N_2O exposure levels in their settings and the ways to minimize trace gas. However, there is evidence that some professionals practice without scavenging equipment and without the use of any other suggested recommendations.[36–38] The use of equipment that does not have scavenging capabilities is clearly a breach of the standard of care.

C. Research continues to surface in the literature regarding the occupational exposure of healthcare practitioners to nitrous oxide. Professionals are taking heed to follow recommended practice protocols and monitor personal exposure. Many articles cite the

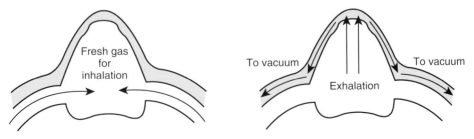

Fresh gas for inhalation

To vacuum   To vacuum

Exhalation

Figure 17-1 Diagram of scavenging nasal hood.

effectiveness of methods to scavenge trace gas, noting dramatic decreases in ppm of N_2O in ambient air.[39-49]

IV. DETECTION AND MONITORING OF N_2O

A. Infrared (IR) spectrophotometry

1. IR spectrophotometry uses electromagnetic energy to detect levels of N_2O in the atmosphere. This technology can detect levels lower than 1 ppm. Figure 17-2 shows an IR spectrophotometer.
2. Other gases can be detected with this technology as well. An advantage of IR spectrophotometry is the ability to detect minute levels of gas immediately in the ambient air.
3. The instrument can be rented for a reasonable fee and used to instantly detect the presence of N_2O in any setting.
4. This method of analyzing trace gas contamination in the environment is recommended to establish a baseline reference of N_2O exposure levels. Depending on the results, low levels may be confirmed because of the use of scavenging methods; high levels indicate the necessity to implement the recommended scavenging methods. Periodic evaluation with this instrument is advised.

B. Time-weighted average (TWA) dosimetry

1. It is also possible to determine the amount of N_2O exposure of an individual over time. This method gives an estimate of the amount of exposure to a gas over a specified period.
2. The badge or vial (similar to a radiation-dosimetry badge) is worn for the recommended period (during exposure or a full workweek) and then returned to the company for analysis. An active material in the badge absorbs the N_2O. The amount is read by an IR spectrophotometer (Figure 17-3) to determine the parts per million of exposure.
3. An advantage to this system is that it is inexpensive and allows for monitoring in a practice that does not extensively use N_2O. Several companies offer these personal monitoring devices. See Appendix A for reference information.

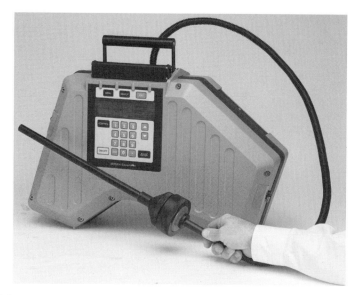

Figure 17-2 Infrared spectrophotometer. *(Courtesy of Thermo Environmental Instruments, Inc., Franklin, Massachusetts.)*

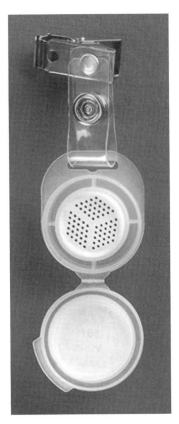

Figure 17-3 Time-weighted average dosimetry badge. *(Courtesy of Assay Technology, Pleasanton, California.)*

C. Hand-held monitoring device (Bacharach N_2O Monitor 3010; new model to be released in late 2007)
   1. An innovative product on the market is a small, lightweight, portable N_2O gas monitor that gives a continuous measure of N_2O in the ambient air (Figure 17-4).
   2. The 8-oz machine that fits in the palm of your hand has both ppm and TWA measurement capabilities that are activated with the touch of a button. The internal sampling pump is zeroed with fresh ambient air and measures N_2O in 5-ppm increments up to a 10,000 ppm maximum. The TWA capability is available in both real time (more than 8 hours) and elapsed time, which begins when the unit is switched on.
   3. The monitor can also be used to detect leaks around equipment. Another beneficial feature is its ability to store data for record keeping and monitoring purposes.
   4. The cost of the unit is not prohibitive and offers a readily available method for assessing occupational risk of exposure to N_2O. See Figure 17-4 and Appendix A for reference information.

V. SCAVENGING N_2O

A. Scavenging N_2O means minimizing trace amounts of the gas before, during, or after use by the patient.

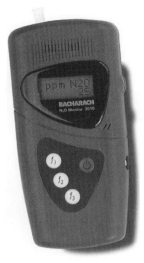

Figure 17-4 Hand-held N_2O monitoring system. *(Courtesy of Bacharach, Inc., Pittsburgh, Pennsylvania.)*

B. The term *scavenging system* traditionally referred to the mask and suction capabilities of the equipment but is currently a term used to identify several methods for the comprehensive removal of trace N_2O.

C. Certain situations are more problematic for scavenging than others.
   1. Patients that are intubated (i.e., tracheal tube) are in a closed-circuit system that affords every opportunity for complete control over trace waste anesthetic gases.
   2. Patients in an ambulatory setting represent a greater opportunity for trace gas loss because of the open circuitry of the sedation machine. N_2O leakage can be found in several places in this setting (Figure 17-5).
   3. Depending on the location of the office (e.g., in a high-rise building), scavenging efforts may be more difficult with regard to ventilation issues.

D. Sources of leakage from the patient
   1. There are several ways that N_2O can leak from the patient. Perhaps the most critical measure to control in this category is patient talking. Whenever patients talk, they are expelling N_2O into the operator's breathing zone. Instruct patients to breathe through their nose and minimize talking.
   2. An ill-fitting mask is a potential source for a significant amount of gas leakage. Ensure a snug, comfortable fit and the appropriate tidal volume before titrating N_2O.
   3. Other leak sources related to the patient are displacement of the mask during patient movement or restlessness, a technical problem with the mask (e.g., a stuck flutter valve), mouth breathing, or a moustache preventing a tight fit.

E. Sources of leakage other than the patient
   1. Gas can leak at any place of connection on the equipment. This includes the manifold and wall-mounted connections and any hoses associated with each.
   2. Conducting tubing and the reservoir bag are areas of concern. Because of the breakdown of some materials, it is possible for these items to crack and subsequently leak around pleats and/or seams (Figure 17-6).
   3. The soap-and-water method (Figure 17-7) for determining leaks is recommended for inspecting the areas mentioned in this section. The presence of bubbles after application of the soap-and-water solution indicates a gas leak. Hand-held devices can also be used (Figure 17-8).

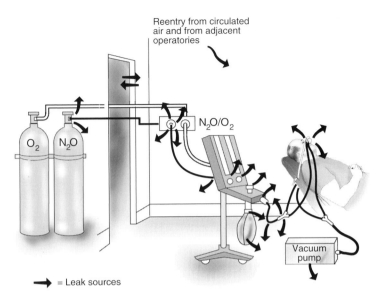

Reentry from circulated
air and from adjacent
operatories

N_2O/O_2

O_2 N_2O

Vacuum
pump

➡ = Leak sources

Figure 17-5 Sources of potential N_2O leaks.

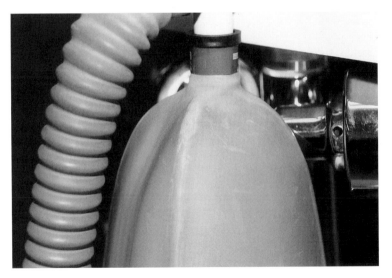

Figure 17-6 N_2O leak potential resulting from the breakdown of certain materials.

4. Door seals and any place where reentry of contaminated air can occur is a potential problem.

F. An evacuation (vacuum) system is used to pull trace gas from the mask into the suction for ultimate dispersal to the outside atmosphere.
   1. Again, the optimal flow rate is 45 L/min.
   2. Adjustment of this suction rate is critical for effective sedation. Too much suction will make the gas unavailable for the patient, and not enough suction will create trace gas contamination by leakage around the mask.
   3. It is important to periodically check this flow rate during sedation.

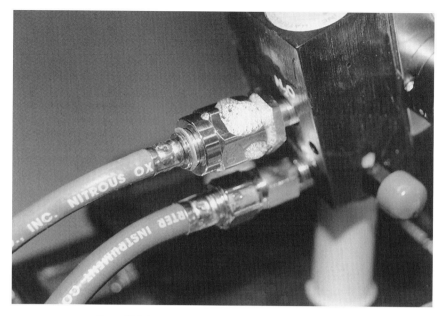

Figure 17-7 Soap and water solution used to test for N_2O leaks.

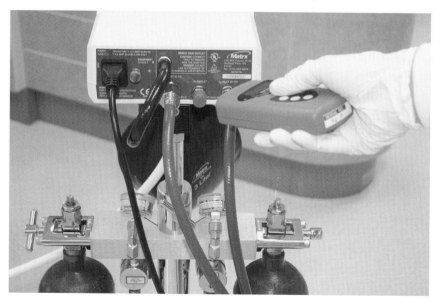

Figure 17-8 Checking connections on the flowmeter for leaks.

G. Adequate ventilation is an area being investigated for improvement.
  1. In a hospital operating room, fresh-air exchange systems are inherent in the design of the room. In an ambulatory setting such as a dental office, there may not be such a provision. Often, air conditioners recirculate ambient air throughout the office, thereby contributing to contamination rather than N_2O elimination. The number of fresh-air exchanges necessary for eliminating trace gas is being investigated.[50]

2. It is recommended that fresh-air inlets be located in the ceiling and designed to direct the fresh-air supply toward the floor to ensure adequate dilution and mixing of the waste gas. Exhaust register louvers should be located near the floor to allow for adequate flushing of the trace N_2O and to prevent short-circuiting of the fresh-air supply.[51]
3. Oscillating room fans can be added to assist in moving the gas to a return vent or to an outside source such as an open window.
4. Monitoring airflow can be accomplished with the use of an electronic micromanometer (Figure 17-9). The AirData Multimeter ADM-850 can detect and measure

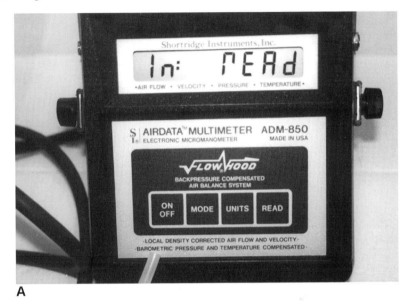

A

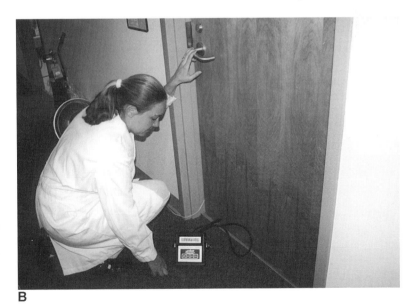

B

Figure 17-9 A and B, Monitoring airflow with an electronic micromanometer.

air velocity, differential pressure, temperature, and airflow. This device is valuable when assessing the adequacy of ventilation in an area. See Figure 17-9 and Appendix A for reference information.

H. Other scavenging strategies

1. Other scavenging devices have been investigated for their ability to assist in minimizing occupational exposure to N_2O and other gases. A combination of increased operatory ventilation and supplemental high-volume aspiration was studied in a laboratory setting for its effect on reducing ambient nitrous oxide levels. The results were positive; however, researchers recognize the limitations of laboratory studies.[52]

2. Local exhaust systems located near the patient's mouth were devised. Noise generated and size of exhaust systems were limitations associated with these devices.[53]

VI. RECOMMENDATIONS AND PREVENTIVE MEASURES

A. Monitor the environment for N_2O concentrations.

1. Establish baseline values if equipment is just being installed. For existing equipment, have the ambient air evaluated periodically with an IR spectrophotometer.

2. Monitor the healthcare professional's personal breathing zone (area immediately adjacent to the nose and mouth in a hemisphere forward of the shoulders with a radius of approximately 18 inches) by use of TWA dosimetry devices.

B. Prevent leakage from the delivery system through proper maintenance and periodic inspection of the equipment.

1. Visually inspect the reservoir bag and conduction tubing for cracks and leaks before each administration.[14]

2. Eliminate or replace loose-fitting connections, loose or deformed slip joints and/or threaded connections, and defective or worn seals or gaskets.

3. Periodically send the sedation equipment back to the manufacturer (depending on their recommendation) for routine evaluation and maintenance. Do not alter, modify, or attempt to adjust this equipment.

C. Control waste N_2O with an appropriate evacuation system that includes securely fitting masks, sufficient evacuation flow rates (45 L/min), and properly vented pumps.

D. Assess the adequacy of room ventilation and air exchange for effectively removing waste N_2O.

1. If concentrations are above 25 ppm but less than 150 ppm, it is recommended to increase exhausting capabilities in the area.[54]

2. Supplement local ventilation to capture the N_2O at the source, add oscillating sweep fans, and/or increase the airflow and air exchange to the room.

E. Institute an education program for members of the healthcare team that describes the hazards of N_2O and defines the preventive measures for reducing or eliminating trace gas contamination (Box 17-1).

VII. SUMMARY

A. N_2O/O_2 sedation is a very valuable tool in the ambulatory health setting for the control of pain and anxiety. Practitioners will continue to rely on its effectiveness.

B. To date, no direct evidence exists of any causal relationship between chronic low-level exposure to N_2O and potential biologic effects. The maximum safe concentration of N_2O has not been determined; however, every attempt should be made to reduce the level of trace N_2O to exposed healthcare personnel. Practitioners cannot be too cautious when their health and that of their coworkers is at stake.

C. Continued research efforts for the scientific advancement of topics related to chronic exposure to N_2O and additional ways to minimize and/or eliminate trace gas

---

Box 17-1 **SUGGESTED OFFICE PROTOCOL**

1. Possess appropriate delivery system with scavenging capabilities, accurate flowmeter, adequate vacuum, and variety of sizes of masks.
2. Assess the adequacy of ventilation system.
   Vent exhaust to outside.
   Provide fresh-air exchange whenever possible.
3. Assess the adequacy of suction system.
   Ensure vacuum at 45 L/min.
   Select appropriate size of mask.
   Establish appropriate tidal volume.
   Discourage patient talking.
4. Assess ambient air for trace gas levels at baseline and periodically thereafter. Periodic personal sampling of personnel should be conducted as well.
5. Assess cylinder attachments, lines, hosing, and reservoir bag for leaks. Use IR spectrophotometer and soap-and-water tests.
6. Calibrate flowmeter(s) every 2 years.

From ADA Council on Scientific Affairs.

contamination are encouraged. Emphasis should be placed on prospective and well-designed studies. Manufacturers should be encouraged to continue their efforts at creating and maintaining effective and efficient equipment.

D. Continuing education should be required of healthcare professionals who use N_2O/O_2 sedation, as should evidence of proper training with state-of-the-art equipment and administration techniques.

REFERENCES

1. Vaisman A: Working conditions in surgery and their effect on the health of anesthesiologists, *Eksp Khir Anesteziol* 3:44, 1967.
2. Cohen EN, Belville JW, Brown BW: Anesthesia, pregnancy and miscarriage: a study of operating room nurses and anesthetists, *Anesthesiology* 35:343, 1971.
3. Cohen EN et al: Occupational disease among operating room personnel: a national study, *Anesthesiology* 41:321, 1974.
4. Cohen EN et al: A survey of anesthetic health hazards among dentists: report of an American Society of Anesthesiologists ad hoc committee on the effects of trace anesthetics on the health of operating room personnel, *JADA* 90:1291, 1975.
5. Cohen EN et al: Occupational disease in dentistry and chronic exposure to trace anesthetic gases, *JADA* 101:21, 1980.
6. Clark MS, Renehan BW, Jeffers BW: Clinical use and potential biohazards of nitrous oxide/oxygen, *Gen Dent* 45:486, 1997.
7. Weinberg CR, Baird DD, Rowland AS: Pitfalls inherent in retrospective time-to-event studies: the example of time to pregnancy, *Stat Med* 12:867, 1993.
8. Bruce DL, Bach MJ, Arbit J: Trace anesthetic effects on perceptual, cognitive, and motor skills, *Anesthesiology* 40:453, 1974.
9. Yagiela JA: Health hazards and nitrous oxide: a time for reappraisal, *Anesth Prog* 38:1, 1991.
10. Bruce DL, Bach MJ: *Trace Effects of Anesthetic Gases on Behavioral Performance of Operating Room Personnel*, HEW publication No (NIOSH) 76–169, Cincinnati, 1976, U.S. Department of Health, Education, and Welfare.
11. Ericson HA, Kallen AB: Hospitalization for miscarriage and delivery outcome among Swedish nurses working in operating rooms in 1973–1978, *Anesth Analg* 64:981, 1985.
12. Hemminke K, Kyyronen P, Lindbohm ML: Spontaneous abortions and malformation in the offspring of nurses exposed to anaesthetic gases, cytostatic drugs, and other potential hazards in hospitals based on registered information of outcome, *J Epidemiol Community Health* 39:141, 1985.

13. Rowland AS *et al*: Reduced fertility among women employed as dental assistants exposed to high levels of nitrous oxide, *N Engl J Med* 327:993, 1992.

14. ADA Council on Scientific Affairs, ADA Council on Dental Practice: Nitrous oxide in the dental office, *JADA* 128:364, 1997.

15. Eger EI II: Fetal injury and abortion associated with occupational exposure to inhaled anesthetics, *J Am Assoc Nurse Anesth* 59:309, 1991.

16. Fujinagra M, Baden JM, Mazze RI: Susceptible period of nitrous oxide teratogenicity in Sprague–Dawley rats, *Teratology* 40:439, 1989.

17. Nunn JF *et al*: Serum methionine and hepatic enzyme activity in anaesthetists exposed to nitrous oxide, *Br J Anaesth* 54:593, 1982.

18. Sweeney B *et al*: Toxicity of bone marrow in dentists exposed to nitrous oxide, *BMJ* 291:567, 1985.

19. Dookun R *et al*: Nitrous oxide: past, present, and future, *SAAD Digest* 14(1–2):13, 1997.

20. Lassen JA *et al*: Treatment of tetanus: severe bone-marrow depression after prolonged nitrous-oxide anaesthesia, *Lancet* 1:527, 1956.

21. Weimann J: Toxicity of nitrous oxide, *Best Pract Res Clin Anaesthesiol* 17(1):47, 2003.

22. Myles PS *et al*: A review of the risks and benefits of nitrous oxide in current anaesthetic practice, *Anaesth Intensive Care* 32:165, 2004.

23. Weisner G *et al*: High-level, but not low-level, occupational exposure to inhaled anesthetics is associated with genotoxicity in the micronucleus assay, *Anesth Analg* 93:118, 2001.

24. Jevtovic-Tordorovic V *et al*: Prolonged exposure to inhalational anesthetic nitrous oxide kills neurons in adult rat brain, *Neuroscience* 122:609, 2003.

25. Burm AG: Occupational hazards of inhalational anaesthetics, *Best Pract Res Clin Anaesthesiol* 17(1):147, 2003.

26. Eger E *et al*: Current status of nitrous oxide, Unpublished research, 2006.

27. Smith I: Nitrous oxide in ambulatory anaesthesia: does it have a place in day surgical anaesthesia or is it just a threat for personnel and the global environment? *Curr Opin Anaesthesiol* 19:592, 2006.

28. Crouch KG, McGlothlin JD, Johnston OE: A long-term study of the development of N_2O controls at a pediatric dental facility, *AIHAJ* 61:753, 2000.

29. Donaldson D, Orr J: A comparison of the effectiveness of nitrous oxide scavenging devices, *J Can Dent Assoc* 55:535, 1989.

30. Certosimo F *et al*: Clinical evaluation of the efficacy of three nitrous oxide scavenging units during dental treatment, *Gen Dent* Sept/Oct:430, 2002.

31. Crouch KG, Johnston OE: Nitrous oxide control in the dental operatory: auxiliary exhaust and mask leakage, design, and scavenging flow rate as factors, *Am Ind Hyg Assoc J* 57:272, 1996.

32. Donaldson D, Grabi J: The efficiency of nitrous oxide scavenging devices in dental offices, *J Can Dent Assoc* 55:541, 1989.

33. Ooi R, Joshi P, Soni N: Nitrous oxide/oxygen analgesia: the performance of the MC mask delivery system, *J R Soc Med* 85:534, 1992.

34. Shafer SM: Face mask scavenging system, *J Oral Maxillofac Surg* 51:945, 1993.

35. Quarnstrom F: Nitrous oxide safety: how safe is it for staff? What can be done to make it safer? *Dent Today* 18 (12):74, 1999.

36. Dunning DG, McFarland K, Safarik M: Nitrous-oxide use. I. Risk of potential exposure and compliance among Nebraska dentists and dental assistants, *Gen Dent* 44:520, 1997.

37. Wilson S: A survey of the American Academy of Pediatric Dentistry membership: nitrous oxide and sedation, *Pediatr Dent* 18:287, 1996.

38. ECRI Reporting System: Hazard update: nitrous oxide cryosurgical units must be scavenged, *Health Devices* 25:306, 1996.

39. Schuyt HC, Verberk MM: Measurement and reduction of nitrous oxide in operating rooms, *Occup Environ Med* 38:1036, 1996.

40. Imberti R, Preseglio I, Imbriani M: Low flow anaesthesia reduces occupational exposure to inhalation anaesthetics, *Acta Anaes Scand* 39:586, 1995.

41. Lucchini R, Toffoletto F, Camerino D: Neurobehavioral functions in operating theatre personnel exposed to anesthetic gases, *Med Lav* 86:27, 1995.

42. Hoerauf KH *et al*: Occupational exposure to sevoflurane and nitrous oxide in operating room personnel, *Int Arch Occup Environ Health* 69:134, 1997.

43. Chang WP, Kau CW, Hseu SS: Exposure of anesthesiologists to nitrous oxide during pediatric anesthesia, *Ind Health* 35:112, 1997.

44. Ahlborg G Jr, Axelsson G, Bodin G: Shift work, nitrous oxide exposure and subfertility among Swedish midwives, *Int J Epidemiol* 25:783, 1996.
45. Breum NO, Kann T: Elimination of waste anaesthetic gases from operating theatres, *Acta Anaesthesiol Scand* 32:388, 1988.
46. Hobbhahn J *et al*: Occupational exposure to sevoflurane, halothane and nitrous oxide during paediatric anaesthesia, *Anaesthesia* 52:215, 1997.
47. Chessor E *et al*: Evaluation of a modified scavenging system to reduce occupational exposure to nitrous oxide in labor and delivery rooms, *J Occup Environ Hyg* 2:314, 2005.
48. Weisner G *et al*: A follow-up study on occupational exposure to inhaled anaesthetics in Eastern European surgeons and circulating nurses, *Int Arch Occup Environ Health* 74:16, 2001.
49. Krenzischek DA *et al*: Phase I collaborative pilot study: waste anesthetic gas levels in the PACU, *J PeriAnesthesia Nursing* 17(4):227, 2002.
50. Borganelli GN, Primosch RE, Henry RJ: Operatory ventilation and scavenger evacuation rate influence on ambient nitrous oxide levels, *J Dent Res* 72:1275, 1993.
51. Howard WR: Nitrous oxide in the dental environment: assessing the risk, reducing the exposure, *JADA* 128:356, 1997.
52. Henry RJ, Borganelli GN: High-volume aspiration as a supplemental scavenging method for reducing ambient nitrous oxide levels in the operatory: a laboratory study, *Int J Paediatr Dent* 5:157, 1995.
53. Byhahn C *et al*: Surgeon's occupational exposure to nitrous oxide and sevoflurane during pediatric surgery, *World J Surg* 25(9):1109, 2001.
54. McGlothlin JD, Crounch KG, Mickelsen RL: *Control of Nitrous Oxide in Dental Operatories*, DHHS No (NIOSH) 94–129, Cincinnati, 1994, U.S. Department of Health and Human Services, Public Health Service, Centers for Disease Control and Prevention, National Institute for Occupational Safety and Health, Division of Physical Sciences and Engineering, Engineering Control Technology Branch.

N₂O Abuse Issues

N₂O has been used for recreational purposes since its discovery in the late eighteenth century. Sir Humphrey Davy and Dr. Gardner Colton traveled extensively proclaiming the exhilarating effects of inhaling N₂O in those early days. Inhaling the gas was popular at social gatherings during that time and is still done at parties today. N₂O abuse is an issue about which everyone should be aware. When chronically abused, N₂O can have serious health ramifications. N₂O should be given the same respect that is given to any drug.

I. INHALANT ABUSE

A. All drugs that produce euphoria have the potential to be abused, whether they are injected, swallowed, or inhaled. However, not all drugs that can be abused through inhalation are defined as "inhalants." The term *inhalant* applies to a group of substances that produce psychoactive reactions and are defined solely by their route of administration.[1] The commonality between these substances is that they are volatile at room temperature, not otherwise defined in another classification, and used to alter consciousness. Typical modes of administration are nasal inhalation called sniffing or snorting, inhaling contents from a bag or bagging, holding a saturated rag in the mouth and inhaling or huffing, and spraying the substance directly into the mouth.[1]

B. Inhalants are generalized to three categories: volatile solvents, nitrites, and N₂O.[2] Solvents are abused much more than nitrites and N₂O.

C. Inhaling chemicals found in a variety of household products is a method of achieving a quick, exhilarating high. It is particularly unfortunate that this type of inhalant abuse seems to be most common among children and adolescents. Statistics have historically appeared in the literature. For example, a survey conducted by the National Institute on Drug Abuse revealed that the number of people 12 years of age and older who admitted to having used inhalants increased dramatically from 1.5 million young persons to more than 18 million users between the years 2000 and 2001.[3] In addition, it was revealed that more 8th graders than high schoolers were using inhalants.[3] Inhalants were second behind marijuana as the most commonly used illicit drugs by teenagers in the 1990s.[4] Studies in the 1980s indicated that 18.6% of U.S. high school seniors had practiced inhaling chemicals at least once; specific states claimed even higher incidence figures and younger users.[5] A 1993 report from the National Institute on Drug Abuse[6] (NIDA) indicates approximately 17% of U.S. adolescents say they have sniffed inhalants. For youth and others who may be disadvantaged financially, inhalants present a way of "getting high" that is cheap and easily obtained.[5] Another alarming statistic involves pregnant women. The National Institute on Drug Abuse reports that 12,000 pregnant women use inhalants each year.[7]

D. These younger users claim a variety of favorite inhalant products. Euphoria-producing chemicals, found in commonly used products, are readily available.

    1. Examples of volatile solvents that are inhaled include fuels such as gasoline, butane, and propane; solvents; paint and paint thinner; rubber cement; airplane glue; hair spray; shoe polish; nail polish remover; deodorants; lubricating cooking sprays; insect repellent; and typewriter correction fluid (Box 18-1). McGarvey *et al* surveyed 285 adolescents and found that the five most frequently inhaled substances were gasoline, refrigerant (Freon), butane, glue, and nitrous oxide.[8]

    2. Typewriter correction fluid is one of the favored inhalants. It contains the chemical 1,1,1-trichloroethane or trichloroethylene. Through 1988, abuse of this substance was responsible for 27 reported fatalities. A leading manufacturer incorporated mustard oil into its product to discourage abuse.[5] Health risks from inhaling this product include liver damage, cranial neuropathy, and cardiac toxicity.[5]

E. Many inhalants are CNS depressants that produce sensations similar to the effects of sedation and anesthesia. However, abusers are looking for the exhilarating, euphoric, visually stimulating effects. Effects are produced in less than 1 minute and are usually not long lasting. Some experienced users claim to feel effects for up to 45 minutes and can, therefore, time their experiences to prolong their exuberance for hours.[5] Disorientation can occur; nausea and vomiting have been reported, as well as sneezing, coughing, and salivation.[9]

F. Obviously, these products are sold legally and are relatively inexpensive. They are found at home and in the garage. They are purchased in grocery, hardware, and drug stores. They can be packaged in small containers that are easily hidden. Most often, purchase of such products causes no suspicion. However, in some areas local sale restrictions may apply.

G. Other risk groups for abuse of these inhalants include those who may be occupationally exposed to the products. Those at risk may be janitors, painters, dry cleaning personnel, automobile repair workers, or hairstylists.[5]

H. Amyl nitrite and butyl nitrite ("poppers") are muscle relaxants inhaled primarily to intensify and prolong sexual experiences. Marketed as room deodorizers, these products may produce symptoms such as headaches, blurred vision, and cardiac arrhythmia.[5]

I. N$_2$O falls into the inhalant classification as well. It has similar pharmacokinetic properties to those products just listed. It is relatively inexpensive, readily accessible, and legal to purchase, and produces a rapid, euphoric high. Users recommend its use to others claiming that it produces feelings of floating or flying; vivid, visual, colorful images; and loss of all inhibitions, making the user feel invincible. Of course, the negative side effects like fatigue, fainting, nausea, and cardiac arrest are rarely mentioned.

J. Death has been associated with inhalant abuse. Death can occur the first time a person inhales a toxic substance. Cardiac dysfunction, respiratory depression, and asphyxiation are the likely causes of death.[10] Suicidal and accidental deaths have also been associated with inhalant abuse. Bowen *et al*[11] reported 52 deaths in Virginia between 1987 and 1996 that were associated with inhalation compounds. Thirty-nine of the deaths resulted from acute voluntary exposure.[11] Victims' ages ranged from 13–42 years, with 19 years being the average age when death occurred.

Box 18-1   **COMMONLY INHALED SUBSTANCES**

Typewriter correction fluid	Hair spray, cooking spray, deodorant spray
Butane, gasoline, propane	Insect repellants
Paint and paint thinner	N$_2$O
Rubber cement, model glue	

II. N₂O ABUSE

A. N$_2$O abusers tend to be somewhat older than those inhaling solvents and fuels, etc. As when it was first introduced, N$_2$O is popular today at college social activities such as parties and concerts and may be advertised in college papers or flyers. N$_2$O etiquette can be found in high-society magazines; reference to its use at elite parties can be found in novels. Now instructions for its use can be found even on the Internet.

B. Healthcare personnel who have ready access to the gas are noted recreational users. In general, health professionals have access to many drugs, and abuse is often not limited to one drug. Anesthesiologists and those in training, students in psychiatric and maxillofacial programs, physicians, and dentists are groups cited in the literature as being substance abusers.[12–15] In a 1977 anonymous survey of medical and dental students, 20% admitted to the use of N$_2$O socially.[16]

C. N$_2$O is easy to obtain for recreational use and is found in several forms.
  1. Because it is commonly found compressed in cylinders and used for medical and dental purposes, it is easy to locate in hospitals, clinics, dental offices, etc.
      a. Several agencies have reported stolen cylinders from such facilities. Individuals employed in such a setting may be able to use the gas on site rather than take the risk of stealing the cylinder.
      b. Distribution centers where cylinders of N$_2$O are filled and distributed to various sites report occasional robbery attempts. Large cylinders previously stored outside of buildings have been moved indoors for security.
  2. N$_2$O is also used in the auto racing industry, since it supports combustion. It is used as an engine-boosting agent. However, N$_2$O used for this purpose is often mixed with sulfur dioxide. Inhaling this noxious mixture is likely to render a person ill with vomiting, headache, and diarrhea, thereby discouraging abuse.
  3. Messina and Wynne,[17] researching homemade N$_2$O, produced the gas according to instructions widely distributed in "head shops" and claimed that the process was easy and inexpensive. They also reported that significant concentrations of nitrogen dioxide and nitric oxide are produced with this method. These substances are toxic and can cause transient pulmonary toxicity and tissue damage.
  4. N$_2$O is approved by the Food and Drug Administration (FDA) as a food ingredient, because the dairy industry uses it as a whipping cream propellant. The gas expands into the cream causing it to whip into foam. When used for these legitimate purposes, N$_2$O is found in 3-inch-long containers called whippets (Figure 18-1). These containers hold approximately 4–5 L of N$_2$O. These products are also misused for recreational purposes.
      a. In addition to the whippet charger, a "cracker" and a balloon is purchased (Figure 18-2). A balloon is attached to one end while the charger is placed

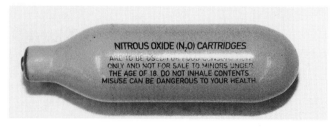

Figure 18-1 Whipping cream charger "whippet."

between the two halves of the cracker. A pointed extension inside the cracker pierces the diaphragm on the charger as the two halves are screwed together. The gas is expelled out of the charger and fills the balloon.

5. Similarly, approximately 3 L of N_2O is found in aerosol cans of whipping cream. It is the N_2O that whips the cream coming out of the can. Figure 18-3 illustrates N_2O listed as a propellant.

   a. This activity becomes a game as users try to "hit" off of a can in a grocery store without buying the product. This "grocery store high" was reported in the psychiatric literature in 1978.[18] Restaurants have reported the necessity of locking the supply of whipping cream cans to prevent restaurant servers from sampling the N_2O while on the job.

   b. To prohibit inhaling N_2O from the aerosol can without purchasing it, manufacturers have considered wrapping the entire can in tamper-resistant plastic.

   c. N_2O can also be found in chargers that are similar in size to a seltzer bottle. Again, the legitimate use is for creating whipped cream; however, those misusing it inhale the contents directly from the bottle or dispel it into balloons.[19]

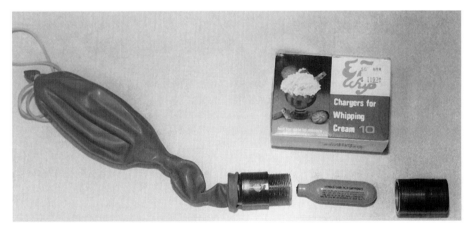

Figure 18-2 Whippet assembly for recreational misuse.

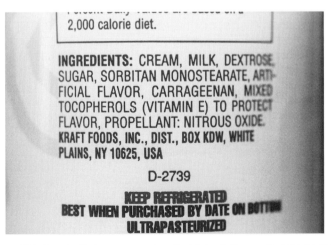

2,000 calorie diet.

INGREDIENTS: CREAM, MILK, DEXTROSE, SUGAR, SORBITAN MONOSTEARATE, ARTI- FICIAL FLAVOR, CARRAGEENAN, MIXED TOCOPHEROLS (VITAMIN E) TO PROTECT FLAVOR, PROPELLANT: NITROUS OXIDE. KRAFT FOODS, INC., DIST., BOX KDW, WHITE PLAINS, NY 10625, USA

D-2739

KEEP REFRIGERATED
BEST WHEN PURCHASED BY DATE ON BOTTLE
ULTRAPASTEURIZED

Figure 18-3 Aerosol whipping cream can ingredient list; note the propellant listed is N₂O.

D. Because of the pharmacokinetics of the drug, N_2O is rarely detected in routine urine tests.[20] Therefore, users may substitute N_2O for other, more detectable drugs, especially when driving. However, there have been reports of youth involved in fatal car accidents when under the influence of N_2O.[19]

III. HEALTH HAZARDS ASSOCIATED WITH CHRONIC EXPOSURE TO N_2O

A. N_2O has been shown to affect vitamin B_{12} metabolism. It oxidizes the cobalt ion in the vitamin B_{12} cofactor, rendering the enzyme methionine synthase inactive in folate metabolic pathways. Methionine synthase plays a vital role in the production of DNA. Megaloblastic hematopoiesis and leukopenia result after prolonged exposure to N_2O.[21]

1. For most healthy surgical or ambulatory patients undergoing N_2O/O_2 sedation, the effects of inactivated methionine synthase are temporary and insignificant. There seems to be a greater risk for pregnant women, those with impaired wound healing capabilities, and for those with existing vitamin B_{12} deficiencies.[21]

2. Studies on laboratory animals have shown that enzyme inactivation occurs rapidly during N_2O overexposure and that recovery is slow.[21,22] Animal studies have also shown evidence of fetal toxicity, resulting in skeletal abnormalities and miscarriages after significant exposure to N_2O in terms of concentration and time.[21]

3. Several studies with humans revealed significant hematopoietic changes as well; the earliest report was cited in 1956.[23–25] Research has confirmed this consequence over the years. An excellent reference list to this subject can be found in Eger's text,[26] *Nitrous Oxide, N_2O.*

4. Individuals who are chronically exposed to N_2O through its recreational use or occupational use in unscavenged areas may be at risk for hematopoietic changes and other sequelae. Chapter 17 provides further details on the biohazard and scavenging issues associated with trace gas contamination.

5. Those persons who are vitamin B_{12} deficient may not be aware of the deficiency until the N_2O exposure produces neurologic changes.[27,28]

   a. Practitioners reveal in the literature instances in which patients with preexisting vitamin B_{12} deficiencies, folate abnormalities, or inherited folate disorders, or those taking antifolate medication may be at risk for adverse effects when exposed to N_2O.[29] A reported case of subacute combined degeneration of the spinal cord occurred postoperatively after surgery with N_2O in a patient found to be vitamin B_{12} deficient.[30] Other citations of myelopathy appear in the literature; many involve prolonged nitrous oxide use.[28,31–34]

   b. It has been suggested that a vitamin B_{12} supplement be taken by women exposed to N_2O as a method for reducing fetotoxic effects.[27] The possibility of biochemical protection exists for other compromised individuals as well. It has been suggested that preoperative concentration levels of vitamin B_{12} be established and deficiencies corrected to avoid possible neurologic complications.[35]

   c. Researchers agree that this is an area in need of continued study.

B. Neurologic side effects have been associated with chronic use of N_2O. Several reports in the literature cite peripheral neuropathy in individuals who indicate habitual use of N_2O.[36]

1. Neurologic symptoms have been reported primarily by individuals who have admitted to the use of N_2O recreationally[37]; however, in some cases, affected individuals were exposed to significant amounts of unscavenged N_2O in hospitals or during dental surgery.[38] Symptoms relating to peripheral neuropathy are evidenced by tingling and numbness in the extremities, weakness and incoordination, lack of strength and

dexterity in the hands, slowed gait, and positive Lhermitte's sign (electric shock feeling on flexion of the neck).[39–41]

2. Often the neuropathic symptoms are not immediate; they may appear several months into the overexposure period.[42] Generally, neurologic function slowly returns to normal after termination of overexposure to the gas. This return is gradual and, in some cases, may not be complete.[42]

3. The cases of overexposure reported in the literature are primarily dentists or other health professionals who deliver N$_2$O to patients without proper scavenging equipment.[32] Other cases are young adults recreationally inhaling N$_2$O from whipping cream chargers.[29,32] Most of the overexposure incidents reported were periods of 1–2 hours per day, at least three times a week, and for periods of several months to years.[27,32] In some cases, individuals reported falling asleep and incurring up to 4 hours of exposure; one individual admitted self-administration of 2–4 hours per day and another admitted 6–7 hours per day.[32]

C. Frostbite has been cited as a consequence of exposure to N$_2$O. An adult male experienced an accident at his place of employment in which a pressure-reducing valve broke from an N$_2$O cylinder, exposing the man to the gas. He was treated for life-threatening pharyngeal swelling from severe frostbite of the oral cavity.[43] More significant are reports of individuals sniffing N$_2$O straight from the cylinder, causing their mouths, lips, and cheeks to freeze to the extent that tissue necrosed to a fourth-degree burn.[44] The temperature of the N$_2$O gas streaming from a cylinder may be as low as $-55°$ C.[33] In one instance, an individual became so disoriented from inhaling the gas that he was unaware that his cheek was in contact with the gas and cylinder for a prolonged period.[44]

D. There have been reports of pneumothorax or pneumomediastinum resulting from the pressure released from a whippet charger. In one instance, actual rupture of alveolar walls occurred, causing interstitial emphysema.[45]

E. Several reports of asphyxial death from N$_2$O are stated in the literature.[46–49] All victims had used N$_2$O recreationally. Several victims have been healthcare workers, others worked in restaurants, and some were users outside of the workplace.

1. The reported deaths of healthcare workers usually involve cylinder apparatus with face masks. Details surrounding the instances reveal victims being found near tanks in healthcare settings.

2. Other reports describe victims being discovered with plastic bags over their heads and belts or similar devices around their necks to keep the bags closed. In these situations, chargers are frequently used and are discharged inside the plastic bag.

   a. Wagner et al[20] recreated the scenario of discharging a whipping cream charger inside a plastic bag. Within 10 seconds of discharging, the 21% O$_2$ concentration found in ambient air inside the bag had dropped to 13%, and the N$_2$O concentration escalated to 59%. Within 1 minute, the O$_2$ concentration had fallen to 10%.

   b. Unconsciousness occurs either from the hypoxia or the drug concentration, and death results when available O$_2$ is depleted to a level that does not support life.[20] Death by this means sometimes may be sought intentionally and other times may be accidental.

3. In one case, N$_2$O was implicated as the cause for an autoerotic asphyxial death. The victim had created a method of delivering N$_2$O through an outdated and modified anesthesia machine, and sexual material describing bondage and other autoerotic methods was found at the scene.[50]

IV. SEXUAL PHENOMENA ASSOCIATED WITH N_2O

A. Euphoric effects have been associated with N_2O since it was first introduced. Some reports in the literature have indicated that hallucinations, visualizations, and auditory illusions have resulted from N_2O abuse.[51] There have also been situations in which aberrations of a sexual nature have been reported.[52]

   1. Allegations of sexual impropriety have been made against health professionals after patients were sedated with N_2O/O_2. These complaints were taken to court for prosecution, but in most cases the charges were dismissed. However, continued licensure was subject to the discretion of the state's licensing board.

   2. Specific cases reported have been primarily against male practitioners by female patients. The cases report claims such as the patient falling asleep and being frightened by a vision, pressure sensations in the genital region, becoming sexually stimulated, feeling naked, dreaming, and fantasizing.[52]

   3. Jastak and Malamed[52] reported that in all of those instances, concentrations of N_2O higher than 50% were used. They also indicated that no other personnel accompanied the dentist during the sedation experience.[52] They recommended that a third party be present at all times and that N_2O concentrations greater than 50% be avoided.

   4. Lambert[53] suggested that hypnosis is potentiated by N_2O. He suggested that a person may experience a hypnotic state spontaneously or by the suggestive language of the professional while N_2O is being administered. Lambert[53] recommended that practitioners regard their statements in a professional manner without lending comments that could be misinterpreted. He recommended suggesting visual imagery such as a beach scene to avoid the patient's own imaging.

B. Obviously, the allegation of sexual impropriety can create uncomfortable situations. Use common sense when N_2O is used; do not place yourself in potentially incriminating situations. Practice with a third party in the vicinity who is educated on the effects of N_2O. Titrate to the appropriate endpoint of sedation to avoid high concentrations of N_2O and oversedation symptoms.

V. ADDICTIVE NATURE OF N_2O

A. Compared with other drugs, N_2O abuse is low.[19] It is not listed among the most commonly abused drugs. This drug has been used for 150 years without mention of significant abuse and addiction problems.

B. Evidence exists that suggests N_2O is involved with the endogenous opioid system directly at a receptor site and/or indirectly by activating opioid neurotransmitters.

   1. Also indicated is the fact that N_2O may be considered a partial opioid agonist, making it less addictive than a full agonist such as morphine.[54]

   2. Autotolerance may be an issue with N_2O, indicating that the body rapidly becomes tolerant to its effects.[20]

C. Compared with other drugs, N_2O abuse does not exist as a public health concern. Alcohol, nicotine, and cannabis have been cited as the most commonly used nonmedical drugs.[55] However, it is still important to be aware of its recreational use among youth and health professionals in particular.

VI. LEGISLATION AND REGULATION ISSUES

A. Currently, there are few regulations governing the sale or purchase of N_2O. Distributors are ethically obligated to confirm that their customers are purchasing the drug for appropriate use; however, there are no control measures to ensure that this is happening. Those selling

N$_2$O for purposes other than appropriate use may be held responsible for their actions. In March 2001, "delivering a misbranded drug into interstate commerce" was the charge that led an Arizona man to 15 months in prison and a fine of $40,000. His sale of N$_2$O in whipped cream chargers led to the death of a college student.[56]

B. Warning labels can be found on cylinders, whippets, and whipping cream containers containing N$_2$O. The labels recommend that users be familiar with the administration and properties of the drug and that misuse could be harmful.

C. The Compressed Gas Association Foundation, the CGA, and the NWSA have been active in informing the public about the concern of N$_2$O misuse. The Nitrous Oxide Abuse Task Force was established in 1994 by the CGA and NWSA. They created the Sales and Security Guidelines for the Safe Use/Handling of Nitrous Oxide.[57] The guidelines provide suggestions and information to producers, repackagers, distributors, carriers, and legitimate users of the gas. Those intended to receive these guidelines range from healthcare and restaurants to auto racing, law enforcement, and trucking. See Appendix A for references to this information.

D. In addition to these guidelines, the CGA and NWSA are working with other organizations to tighten distribution policies and develop strong codes of ethics for voluntary implementation. They also provide assistance to those working with law enforcement individuals dealing with N$_2$O misuse issues.

E. Legislatively, these organizations have been instrumental in assisting the development of model state legislation that would discourage illicit N$_2$O use by prohibiting unlawful possession and/or distribution. Violations are punishable by law. Several states in the United States have been on the forefront of this issue and have already been successful in enacting legal regulations. There are states with specific laws against the sale of nitrous oxide. Those states are Arizona, Connecticut, Florida, Louisiana, Maryland, Michigan, Ohio, West Virginia, and Wisconsin. Other states that have laws prohibiting the sale of intoxicants are Illinois, Kentucky, New Hampshire, and North Carolina. It is likely that the sale of nitrous oxide could be cited in these states. Several states specifically name nitrous oxide in laws prohibiting the possession of inhalants. Those states are California, Georgia, Iowa, North Carolina, and Oregon. In addition, states in which inhaling is unlawful are Colorado, Hawaii, Massachusetts, Maine, Minnesota, Nebraska, Nevada, Rhode Island, Texas Utah, Virginia, and Vermont. The Florida law makes it illegal for any person to possess, distribute, or sell more than 16 grams of N$_2$O. Perpetrators are charged with a third-degree felony and could be required to participate in a substance abuse program.[58] These states are to be commended for their involvement in the control of illicit N$_2$O use.

REFERENCES

1. Brouette T, Anton R: Clinical review of inhalants, *Am J Addictions* 10:79, 2001.
2. Weir E: Inhalant use and addiction in Canada, *CMAJ* 164(3):397, 2001.
3. Office of Applied Studies: *Results from the 2000 and 2001 National Household Survey on Drug Abuse*: *Volume I and III. Summary of National Findings*, DHHS Publication numbers SMA 01–3549 and SMA 02–3758, Rockville, 2000–2002, Substance Abuse and Mental Health Services Administration, National Clearinghouse for Alcohol and Drug Information.
4. Edwards RW, Oetting ER: Inhalant use in the United States, *Natl Inst Drug Abuse Res Monogr Ser* 148:8, 1995.
5. Schwartz RJ: When to suspect inhalant abuse, *Patient Care* 30:39, 1989.
6. National Institute on Drug Abuse Website: www.nida.nih.gov.
7. Jones HE, Balster RL: Inhalant abuse in pregnancy, *Obstet Gynecol Clin North Am* 25(1):153, 1998.
8. McGarvey EL *et al*: Adolescent inhalant abuse: environments of use, *Am J Drug Alcohol Abuse* 25(4):731, 1999.
9. McHugh MJ: The abuse of volatile substances, *Pediatr Clin North Am* 34:333, 1987.

10. Adgey AA, Johnston PW, McMechan S: Sudden cardiac death and substance abuse, *Resuscitation* 29(3):219, 1995.
11. Bowen SE *et al:* Deaths associated with inhalant abuse in Virginia from 1987 to 1996, *Drug Alcohol Depend* 53:239, 1999.
12. Gillman MA: Nitrous oxide abuse in perspective, *Clin Neuropharmacol* 15:297, 1992.
13. From RP: Substance dependence and abuse by anesthesia care providers. In Rogers M *et al*, editors: *Principles and Practice of Anesthesiology*, St. Louis, 1993, Mosby.
14. Kenna GA, Wood MD: The prevalence of alcohol, cigarette and illicit drug use and problems among dentists, *JADA* 136:1023, 2005.
15. Seidberg BH, Sullivan TH: Dentists' use, misuse, abuse or dependence on mood-altering substances, *NYSDJ* April:30, 2004.
16. Rosenberg H, Orkin FK, Springstead J: Abuse of nitrous oxide, *Anesth Analg* 58:104, 1979.
17. Messina FV, Wynne JW: Homemade nitrous oxide: no laughing matter, *Ann Intern Med* 96:333, 1982.
18. Block SH: The grocery store high, *Am J Psychiatry* 135:126, 1978.
19. Murray MJ, Murray WJ: Nitrous oxide availability, *J Clin Pharm* 20:202, 1980.
20. Wagner SA *et al:* Asphyxial deaths from the recreational use of nitrous oxide, *J Forensic Sci* 37:1008, 1992.
21. Nunn JF, Chanarin I: Nitrous oxide inactivates methionine synthetase. In Eger EI II: *Nitrous Oxide N$_2$O*, New York, 1985, Elsevier Science Publishing.
22. Londo H, Osborne ML: Nitrous oxide has multiple deleterious effects on cobalamin metabolism and causes decreases in activities of mammalian cobalamin dependent enzymes, *J Clin Invest* 67:1270, 1981.
23. Lassen JC *et al:* Treatment of tetanus: severe bone marrow depression after prolonged nitrous-oxide anaesthesia, *Lancet* 1:527, 1956.
24. Amess JA *et al:* Megaloblastic haemopoiesis in patients receiving nitrous oxide, *Lancet* 2:339, 1978.
25. Skacel PO *et al:* Studies on the haemopoietic toxicity of nitrous oxide in man, *Br J Haematol* 53:189, 1983.
26. Eger EI II: *Nitrous Oxide, N$_2$O*, New York, 1985, Elsevier Science Publishing.
27. Ostreicher JS: Vitamin B$_{12}$ supplements as protection against nitrous oxide inhalation, *NY State Dent J* 60:47, 1994.
28. Butzkueven H, King JO: Nitrous oxide myelopathy in an abuser of whipped cream bulbs, *J Clin Neurosci* 7 (1):73, 2000.
29. Wyatt SS, Gill RS: An absolute contraindication to nitrous oxide, *Anaesthesia* 54(3):307, 1999.
30. Beltramello A *et al:* Subacute combined degeneration of the spinal cord, *J Neurol Neurosurg Psychiatry* 64 (4):563, 1998.
31. Vishnubhakat SM, Beresford HR: Reversible myeloneuropathy of nitrous oxide abuse: serial electrophysiological studies, *Muscle Nerve* 14:22, 1991.
32. Waclawik AJ *et al:* Myeloneuropathy from nitrous oxide abuse: unusually high methylmalonic acid and homocysteine levels, *Wisc Med J* 102(4):43, 2003.
33. Brett A: Myeloneuropathy from whipped cream bulbs presenting as conversion disorder, *Aust NZ J Psychiatry* 31:131, 1997.
34. Alderman CJ, Nyfort-Hansen K: Nitrous oxide abuse in a community setting: case report, *Aust J Hosp Pharm* 30:109, 2000.
35. Mayall M: Vitamin B$_{12}$ deficiency and nitrous oxide, *Lancet* 352(9163):1529, 1999.
36. Kunkel DB: The toxic emergency, *Emerg Med* 19:79, 1987.
37. Iwata K *et al:* Neurologic problems associated with chronic nitrous oxide abuse in a non-healthcare worker, *Am J Med Sci* 322(3):173, 2001.
38. Layzer RB: Myeloneuropathy after prolonged exposure to nitrous oxide, *Lancet* 2:1227, 1978.
39. Sahenk Z *et al:* Polyneuropathy from inhalation of N$_2$O cartridges through a whipped-cream dispenser, *Neurology* 28:485, 1978.
40. Layzer RB, Fishman RA, Schafer JA: Neuropathy following abuse of nitrous oxide, *Neurology* 28:504, 1978.
41. Paulson GW: "Recreational" misuse of nitrous oxide, *JADA* 98:410, 1979.
42. Gutmann L, Johnsen D: Nitrous oxide-induced myeloneuropathy: report of cases, *JADA* 103:239, 1981.
43. Svartling N *et al:* Life-threatening airway obstruction from nitrous oxide induced frostbite of the oral cavity, *Anaesth Intensive Care* 24(6):717, 1996.
44. Hwang JC, Himel HN, Edlich RF: Frostbite of the face after recreational misuse of nitrous oxide, *Burns* 22:152, 1996.
45. LiPuma JP, Wellman J, Stern HP: Nitrous oxide abuse: a new cause for pneumomediastinum, *Radiology* 145:602, 1982.

46. Suruda AJ, McGlothlin JD: Fatal abuse of nitrous oxide in the workplace, *J Occup Med* 32:682, 1990.

47. Garriott J, Petty CS: Death from inhalant abuse: toxicological and pathological evaluation of 34 cases, *Clin Toxicol* 16:305, 1980.

48. Chadly A, Marc B, Barres D: Suicide by nitrous oxide poisoning, *Am J For Med Pathol* 10:330, 1989.

49. Winek CL, Wahba WW, Rozin L: Accidental death by nitrous oxide inhalation, *Forensic Sci Int* 73:139, 1995.

50. Leadbeatter S: Dental anesthetic death: an unusual autoerotic episode, *Am J For Med Pathol* 9:60, 1988.

51. Steinberg H: Abnormal behavior induced by nitrous oxide, *Br J Psychol* 47:183, 1956.

52. Jastak JT, Malamed SF: Nitrous oxide sedation and sexual phenomena, *JADA* 101:38, 1980.

53. Lambert C: Sexual phenomena hypnosis and nitrous oxide sedation, *JADA* 101:990, 1982.

54. Gillman MA: Nitrous oxide, an opioid addictive agent, *Am J Med* 81:97, 1986.

55. Kreek MJ: Multiple drug abuse patterns and medical consequences. In Meltzer HY, editor: *Psychopharmacology: The Third Generation of Progress*, New York, 1987, Raven Press.

56. Meadows M Arizona man sentenced for selling nitrous oxide, *FDA Consumer* May–June: 33, 2001.

57. Compressed Gas Association: *Nitrous Oxide Sales and Security Recommended Guidelines*, Arlington, Va, 2003, Compressed Gas Association.

58. Tuck MG: Law ups ante on nitrous oxide possession and distribution, *J Dent Technol* 17(7):34, 2000.

SUGGESTED READINGS

Dohrn CS *et al:* Reinforcing effects of extended inhalation of nitrous oxide in humans, *Drug Alcohol Depend* 31:265, 1993.

Dzoljic M *et al:* Behavioral and electrophysiological aspects of nitrous oxide dependence, *Brain Res Bull* 33:25, 1994.

Pollard TG: Relative addiction potential of major centrally-active drugs and drug classes—inhalants and anesthetics, *Adv Alcohol Subst Abuse* 9:149, 1990.

Chapter 19

Ethical and Legal Considerations Regarding N₂O Administration

Healthcare professionals are ethically and legally responsible for providing the best care that is possible for each patient. Practitioners are also required to abide by the laws and rules governing their discipline in their area (e.g., state, province, or country). It is vitally important to be educated on all aspects of N_2O/O_2 sedation and be legally certified or licensed by a governing agency when necessary. As stated previously in this text, it is imperative to follow the ASA Practice Guidelines for Sedation and Analgesia by Non-anesthesiologists, because these will be the standards to which your actions will be compared should legal and/or ethical concerns be expressed.

I. LEGAL REQUIREMENTS ASSOCIATED WITH N₂O/O₂ ADMINISTRATION

A. Depending on the discipline and the governing body regulating the requirements of practice within the discipline, there are rules to abide by regarding the administration of N_2O/O_2 sedation.
   1. Widespread variations exist among disciplines as to who may administer and/or monitor the N_2O/O_2 sedation procedure; the licensing agency of the discipline will determine who is or is not eligible to provide this type of service and under what conditions it may be administered. These parameters of practice are monitored by the appropriate governing agency, whose purpose is to protect the public.
      a. Depending on the discipline, a practitioner may only be legally allowed to monitor a patient under N_2O/O_2 sedation and not be allowed to administer the drug. This prohibits the individual from titrating N_2O to the patient. This may be the case for certain levels of auxiliaries within a discipline (Figures 19-1 and 19-2).*
   2. In addition, the law outlines the level of supervision necessary for this procedure. In dentistry, states that allow auxiliaries such as dental hygienists to administer N_2O require that the procedure be under the direct supervision of a dentist.
B. Because so many legal variations of rules that are discipline specific exist, it is critical to be informed of the codified law and administrative rules applicable within each state and then practice only within the scope of that law.
C. It is also legally mandated that informed consent be obtained from the patient or parent or guardian before the administration of N_2O/O_2 sedation. The purpose of informed consent is to respect the patient's right to autonomy and allow him or her the opportunity to make educated decisions about his or her healthcare.
   1. In some states, written consent is required. However, even if not mandated, obtaining a patient's or parent/guardian's signature is advised.

---

*Disclaimer: Always check with the licensing agency of the state in which you practice for the most current and accurate regulations regarding the administration and/or monitoring of N_2O/O_2 sedation.

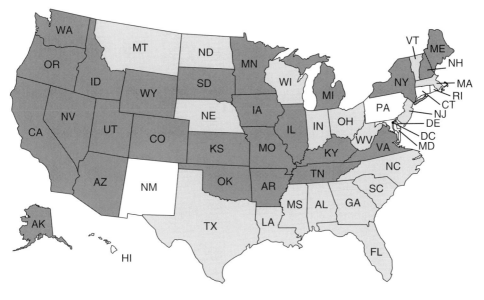

States where dental hygienists can administer nitrous oxide/oxygen sedation

States where dental hygienists can assist in the administration or monitor nitrous oxide/oxygen sedation

States where dental hygienists are not permitted to administer, assist in the administration, or monitor nitrous oxide/oxygen sedation

Figure 19-1 States that allow dental hygienists to administer N$_2$O/O$_2$ sedation.

2. Components of informed consent include patient identification, proposed treatment along with alternatives, and associated costs of that treatment. In addition, risks and potential adverse outcomes are included.
3. With N$_2$O/O$_2$ sedation, it is important that the patient and/or parent/guardian understand why this procedure is being recommended and what can be expected. The patient/parent/guardian must have the opportunity to ask questions, and it is even more important that all his or her questions have been answered.[1]
4. It is prudent practice to confirm the acquisition of informed consent with a patient's or parent's signature at each visit. An example of an appropriate informed consent form for N$_2$O/O$_2$ sedation can be found in Appendix D.

II. APPROPRIATE EDUCATION FOR N$_2$O/O$_2$ ADMINISTRATION

A. Governing boards and licensing agencies may require a specified course of training in the area of N$_2$O/O$_2$ sedation before practitioners can incorporate this procedure into their clinical practices.
1. Often, proof of successful completion of an approved course on the subject is required. Approved courses usually consist of both didactic and clinical components, totaling a specified minimum number of hours.
2. After successful completion of such a course of study and probable fee payment, the practitioner may be granted a permit or license to administer N$_2$O/O$_2$ sedation.

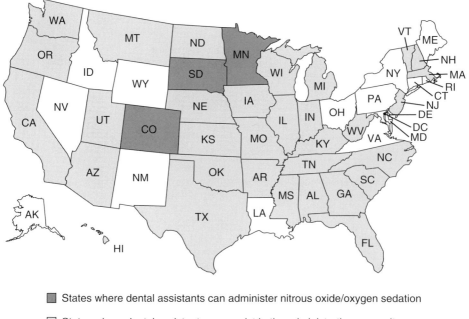

Figure **19-2** States that allow dental assistants to administer or monitor N_2O/O_2 sedation.

3. Most often, students completing their professional curriculum are exempt from additional coursework in this area unless this information was not part of the professional program. In such a case, the student is subject to the same requirements as those without the necessary education.

B. It may be favorable for a previously educated practitioner to participate in an N_2O/O_2 sedation refresher course. Updated material, new equipment, or a review of the appropriate administration technique may be presented, which could enhance the success of this procedure in clinical practice. We have found that those practitioners participating in review courses return to their practices with a renewed appreciation for the drug and its potential. They value the reinforcement of how the procedure is making their practice successful while providing a valuable service to their patients.

III. ETHICAL RESPONSIBILITIES

A. In addition to legal practice guidelines for administering N_2O/O_2 sedation, there are ethical aspects to consider. All health disciplines have a code of ethics through which they inform the public and affirm to their constituents their standards of practice. Each of these codes states that it is the intention of the discipline to uphold high ethical standards for all patients. N_2O/O_2 sedation is available for reducing a patient's pain and anxiety before performing a clinical procedure. It is unethical for a healthcare professional to knowingly administer N_2O to a patient for any other reason (e.g., thrill seeking).

B. The abuse potential of N_2O has been discussed (see Chapter 18). It is the responsibility of the practitioner to ensure that tanks are properly stored and locked securely so that the likelihood of others stealing a tank or abusing N_2O is minimized.

C. **Do not abuse N_2O yourself.** There are significant health risks and complications that could affect you permanently. Seek help if necessary. Also, assist others if you suspect or recognize that they may have a problem.

D. Administer N_2O/O_2 with the recommended titration technique. Use updated, state-of-the-art equipment provided by the manufacturers, because the delivery systems currently available undergo stringent quality control and safety measures.[2] Use recommended scavenging techniques and procedures for minimizing trace gas contamination to exposed personnel (see Chapter 17).

IV. PRACTICE GUIDELINES

A. **Avoid allegations of sexual misconduct.** The propensity exists for a patient to become sexually stimulated or dream or hallucinate sexual situations while sedated with N_2O. Allegations of sexual misconduct can be avoided in obvious ways. Common sense is all that is necessary in most cases.

   1. Use the appropriate technique and titrate to the exact level of appropriate sedation. Most patients achieve this endpoint at N_2O concentrations less than 50%. If the patient requires a percentage higher than 50%, the operator should be alerted to the fact that cumulative effects of the drug may quickly change the level of sedation and that this range is considered high risk for dreaming or fantasizing.

   2. Always have a third party in the room during the procedure as a witness against false accusations.[1]

   3. Do not place yourself in a potentially incriminating situation, such as an after-hours appointment where intentions may be misinterpreted.

B. Be meticulous about record keeping and documentation procedures. Record the details of each sedation experience for every patient in the treatment file.

C. Practice within the standard of care established by the profession. Use updated equipment with the O_2 fail-safe mechanism for safe delivery to the patient. Follow the steps for appropriate N_2O/O_2 administration using the method of titration. Use the recommended scavenging procedures for the sake of those exposed to trace gas contamination.

D. Be knowledgeable about the levels of sedation and be appropriately prepared to handle the next (deeper) level beyond which you have intended. N_2O is a safe drug, but it is your responsibility to know how to react in any given situation.

E. Maintain an adequate and current malpractice insurance policy.

F. Practice within the parameters of the discipline. Do not ask others to perform the procedure when they are not legally allowed to do so, and do not perform the task yourself if you are not permitted.

REFERENCES

1. American Academy of Pediatric Dentistry, Council on Clinical Affairs: *Guideline on Informed Consent*, Chicago, 2005, American Academy of Pediatric Dentistry.
2. American Dental Association: *Guidelines for the Use of Conscious Sedation, Deep Sedation and General Anesthesia for Dentists*, Chicago, 2002, American Dental Association.

Chapter 20

Commonly Asked Questions Regarding N₂O/O₂ Sedation

1. *Can I use oral premedication with N_2O/O_2?*
   Yes, but remember there will be a synergistic effect between the N_2O and other drugs. Therefore, it is important to know the pharmacology of all the drugs involved. You are responsible for all the drugs you administer, and you must be prepared to rescue a patient from the next level of sedation beyond that which was intended.

2. *Is it okay to eat before receiving N_2O/O_2?*
   Yes, a light, nonfatty meal eaten no sooner than 2 hours before the procedure is fine. It is best to avoid heavy meals.

3. *Are there any latex-free products available?*
   Yes, all currently manufactured products are latex free.

4. *Is a pulse oximeter necessary for N_2O/O_2 sedation?*
   No, not if it is given in concentrations below 50%. Above this level, it is recommended to monitor the patient with a pulse oximeter, because that enters the level of moderate sedation.

5. *Is sickle cell anemia a contraindication to N_2O/O_2 use?*
   No, in fact, preventive measures for sickle cell crisis use 100% O_2.

6. *Does the conduction tubing need to be sterilized after each patient?*
   Any part of the tubing that is not corrugated can be sterilized. This can be done after each patient, but it is not necessary. Surface disinfection is adequate.

7. *Can N_2O/O_2 sedation be used in combination with other drugs to enhance sedation?*
   Caution should be given to these situations because the synergistic effect is hard to predict.

8. *How does N_2O affect the lactating (nursing) mother?*
   N_2O has no effect on breast milk.

9. *Can N_2O/O_2 enhance difficult venipuncture?*
   Yes, a short course of N_2O/O_2 can enhance venous distention and visibility.

10. *Can I go back to work right after I've used N_2O?*
    Yes, there is a full and complete recovery after an adequate amount of 100% O_2 after a procedure.

11. *Can I use N_2O without O_2?*
    No, the O_2 molecule must be available for human metabolism. The use of N_2O without O_2 could result in death.

12. *What is the youngest age in which N$_2$O/O$_2$ sedation can be administered?*
    N$_2$O/O$_2$ sedation can be used for patients of any age.

13. *Does insurance pay for N$_2$O/O$_2$ sedation?*
    Yes, some companies reimburse for this service, although others do not. In the United States, the ADA reimbursement code is #09230.

14. *Can a person with asthma use N$_2$O/O$_2$ sedation?*
    Absolutely, asthmatics do very well with N$_2$O.

15. *What is the number one potential negative side effect?*
    Nausea and vomiting. This can occur with an inappropriate administration technique or inadequate monitoring and if inappropriately high concentrations of N$_2$O are used.

16. *Can N$_2$O be used with a laser present?*
    Yes, this is not a contraindication for its use.

17. *Can a rash around the nose indicate an allergy to the nosepiece if it was latex?*
    Yes, if the individual is latex sensitive or if the nasal hood was inappropriately disinfected and not sterilized.

18. *Is it necessary to document the N$_2$O/O$_2$ procedure in the chart?*
    Yes, for legal reasons it is required to document each N$_2$O/O$_2$ procedure. A sample of a sedation record is included in Chapter 13 and in Appendix C.

19. *Where can I rent an infrared (IR) spectrophotometer to measure trace gas N$_2$O in my office?*
    An inexpensive and convenient way is to contact your local hospital or gas supplier.

20. *Is N$_2$O/O$_2$ sedation contraindicated for an individual with congenital birth defects?*
    No. N$_2$O/O$_2$ sedation is used for a variety of medically compromised patients. However, administration depends on the individual's level of understanding no matter what the medical condition.

21. *Is a backup portable system necessary?*
    It is highly recommended to have a second tank of each gas immediately available should one be emptied in the middle of a procedure.

22. *Can you give oxycodone (Vicodin) with N$_2$O/O$_2$ sedation?*
    When the patient is completely recovered from N$_2$O/O$_2$ sedation, any postoperative medication will have no interaction with the previous N$_2$O/O$_2$ experience.

23. *Is there a time limit that a practitioner should be cognizant of when administering N$_2$O/O$_2$ sedation?*
    Although there is no specific time unit, the authors consider 3 hours as an extended time period.

24. *Is a written consent form necessary?*
    Certainly verbal consent must be obtained before each N$_2$O/O$_2$ procedure, and written consent is prudent practice. A sample written consent form has been provided in Appendix D.

25. *Why is the N$_2$O/O$_2$ machine such an important piece of emergency equipment?*
    N$_2$O/O$_2$ sedation machines allow for positive-pressure O$_2$ to be delivered to the patient. This is the treatment for laryngospasm and ensuring the lungs are well ventilated with O$_2$. It also does not require the skill associated with the use of an Ambu bag.

26. *Do you need to titrate the nitrous oxide down when you are finishing with a procedure and getting ready to give 100% oxygen?*
No, it is not necessary to slowly remove the nitrous oxide at the completion of the procedure. Terminate the nitrous oxide flow completely and begin the minimum 5 minutes of postoperative oxygenation.

Future Trends in N$_2$O/O$_2$ Sedation

The future of N$_2$O/O$_2$ sedation has never been brighter. The consumption and use of N$_2$O and O$_2$ for patient management has continued to increase since the last edition of this text. There is substantial demand for continuing education courses both within and outside the United States from a variety of disciplines. In addition to frequent, sizable courses provided by the authors, the Porter Instrument Company has initiated a series of courses throughout the United States for dentists, dental hygienists, and dental assistants as a result of the increased demand and expanding state dental practice acts.

At this time, registered nurses in the United States are now petitioning their state licensing agencies for the privilege to administer N$_2$O/O$_2$ sedation, particularly in the pediatric and emergency departments of the hospital. This new initiative is easily supported by the incredible safety record that N$_2$O possesses and the fact that this information can be easily incorporated into nursing education.

Each of the three major manufacturers of N$_2$O/O$_2$ sedation equipment in the United States—Accutron Inc., Matrx by Midmark, and the Porter Instrument Co.—have made major advancements in their product designs that make simpler, more ergonomic, and state-of-the-art sedation delivery possible. New designs and products have been recently introduced into the market for your use.

In 2006, N$_2$O/O$_2$ sedation was introduced to mainland China by the author. On return visits, this form of sedation was presented to opinion leaders and hospital directors in major cities throughout the country. The introduction of this type of sedation to one quarter of the world's population is truly an unparalleled experience. With the spectacular growth of China's population, the use of N$_2$O/O$_2$ is poised to provide sedative benefits to millions of patients well into the future.

We are delighted to be a part of such a bright future. We know N$_2$O/O$_2$ sedation will continue to play a major role in the relief of patients' pain and anxiety. As the world's population continues to benefit from the advancement of medical science, we will live longer and demand additional health services. N$_2$O/O$_2$ sedation will remain a vital component of patient care well into the future.

Manufacturers and Organizational Resources

AUTHORS

Morris S. Clark, DDS, FACD
University of Colorado School of Dental Medicine
Department of Surgical Dentistry
MS-F847
P.O. Box 6508
13065 E. 17th Ave
Aurora, CO 80045
Telephone: 303-724-6975
Fax: 303-724-6986
Morris.Clark@uchsc.edu

Ann L. Brunick, RDH, MS
Department of Dental Hygiene
University of South Dakota
120 East Hall
414 East Clark Street
Vermillion, SD 57069
Telephone: 605-677-5580
Fax: 605-677-5638
Ann.Brunick@usd.edu

N_2O/O_2 EQUIPMENT MANUFACTURERS (USA)

Accutron, Inc.
1733 Parkside Lane
Phoenix, AZ 85027
Telephone: 800-531-2221
Fax: 602-780-0444
accutron-inc.com

Matrx by Midmark, Inc.
145 Med County Drive
Orchard Park, NY 14127
Telephone: 800-847-1000
Fax: 716-662-8440
matrxmedical.com

Porter Instrument Co., Inc.—A Division of Parker Hannifin
245 Township Line Road, Box 907
Hatfield, PA 19440-0907
Telephone: 215-723-4000
Fax: 215-723-2199
porterinst.com

PERSONAL MONITORING DEVICES
Advanced Chemical Sensor, Inc.
3201 North Dixie Highway
Boca Raton, FL 33431
Telephone: 561-338-3116
Fax: 561-338-5737
advancedchemicalsensors.com

Assay Technology
1252 Quarry Lane
Pleasanton, CA 94566
Telephone: 800-833-1258
Fax: 925-461-7149
assaytec.com

Kem Medical Products Corp.
75 Price Parkway
Farmingdale, NY 11735
Telephone: 800-553-0330
Fax: 631-454-8083
kemmed.com

Medical Safety Systems, Inc.
565 White Pond Drive, Suite E
Akron, OH 44320
Telephone: 888-803-9303
Fax: 330-865-4393
ms2info.com

Nevin Laboratories, Inc.
5000 South Halsted Street
Chicago, IL 60609
Telephone: 800-544-5337
Fax: 773-624-7337
nevinlabs.com

IR SPECTROPHOTOMETRY
Bacharach, Inc.
621 Hunt Valley Circle
New Kensington, PA 15068-7074
Telephone: 800-736-4666 US
Fax: 724-334-5001
bacharach-inc.com

Thermo Electron Corp.
27 Forge Parkway
Franklin, MA 02038
Telephone: 508-553-6861
Fax: 508-520-1460
thermo.com

ELECTRONIC MICROMANOMETER

Shortridge Instruments, Inc.
7855 East Redfield Road
Scottsdale, AZ 85260
Telephone: 480-991-6744
Fax: 480-443-1267
shortridge.com

ORGANIZATIONAL RESOURCES

American Conference of Government Industrial Hygienists
1330 Kemper Meadow Drive, Suite 600
Cincinnati, OH 45240
Telephone: 513-742-2020
Fax: 513-742-3355
acgih.org

American Dental Association
211 East Chicago Avenue
Chicago, IL 60611
Telephone: 800-621-8099
Fax: 312-440-7494
ada.org

American Dental Hygienists' Association
444 North Michigan Avenue, Suite 3400
Chicago, IL 60611
Telephone: 312-440-8900
Fax: 312-440-8929
adha.org

American Dental Society of Anesthesiology
211 East Chicago Avenue, Suite 780
Chicago, IL 60611
Telephone: 877-255-3742
Fax: 312-642-9713
adsahome.org

American Medical Association
515 North State Street
Chicago, IL 60611
Telephone: 800-621-8335
Fax: 312-464-4184
ama-assn.org

American Society of Anesthesiologists
520 North Northwest Highway
Park Ridge, IL 60068-2573
Telephone: 847-825-5586
Fax: 847-825-1692
asahq.org

Centers for Disease Control and Prevention (CDC)
1600 Clifton Road Northeast
Atlanta, GA 30333
Telephone: 800-311-3435
cdc.gov

Compressed Gas Association, Inc.
4221 Walney Road, Fifth Floor
Chantilly, VA 20151-2923
Telephone: 703-788-2700
Fax: 703-961-1831
cganet.com

Gases and Welding Distributors Association
100 North 20th Street, 4th floor
Philadelphia, PA 19103
Telephone: 215-564-3484
Fax: 215-963-9785
gawda.org

National Fire Protection Association
1 Batterymarch Park
Quincy, MA 02169-7471
Telephone: 617-770-3000
Fax: 617-770-0700
nfpa.org

National Inspection Testing Certification (ITC)
501 Shatto Place, Suite 201
Los Angeles, CA 90020
Telephone: 877-457-6482
Fax: 213-382-2501
nationalitc.com

National Institute for Occupational Safety and Health (NIOSH)
4676 Columbia Parkway
Cincinnati, OH 45226
Telephone: 800-356-4674
Fax: 513-533-8573
cdc.gov/niosh

Occupational Safety and Health Administration (OSHA)
Health Standards Programs
United States Department of Labor
200 Constitution Avenue Northwest
Washington, DC 20210
Telephone: 800-321-6742
osha.gov

Piping, Industry, Progress, and Education (PIPE)
501 Shatto Place, Suite 200
Los Angeles, CA 90020
Telephone: 800-457-7473
Fax: 213-382-2501
pipe.org

Percent of N$_2$O/O$_2$ Administered*

Liters per minute N$_2$O	0.5	1	1.5	2	2.5	3	3.5	4	4.5	5	5.5
0.5	50%	33%	25%	20%	17%	14%	13%	11%	10%	9%	8%
1	67%	50%	40%	33%	29%	25%	22%	20%	18%	17%	15%
1.5	75%	60%	50%	43%	38%	33%	30%	27%	25%	23%	21%
2	80%	67%	57%	50%	44%	40%	36%	33%	31%	29%	27%
2.5	83%	71%	63%	56%	50%	45%	42%	38%	36%	33%	31%
3	86%	75%	67%	60%	55%	50%	46%	43%	40%	38%	35%
3.5	88%	78%	70%	64%	58%	54%	50%	47%	44%	41%	39%
4	89%	80%	73%	67%	62%	57%	53%	50%	47%	44%	42%
4.5	90%	82%	75%	69%	64%	60%	56%	53%	50%	47%	45%
5	91%	83%	77%	71%	67%	63%	59%	56%	53%	50%	48%
5.5	92%	85%	79%	73%	69%	65%	61%	58%	55%	52%	50%
6	92%	86%	80%	75%	71%	67%	63%	60%	57%	55%	52%
6.5	93%	87%	81%	76%	72%	68%	65%	62%	59%	57%	54%
7	93%	88%	82%	78%	74%	70%	67%	64%	61%	58%	56%
7.5	94%	88%	83%	79%	75%	71%	68%	65%	63%	60%	58%
8	94%	89%	84%	80%	76%	73%	70%	67%	64%	62%	59%
8.5	94%	89%	85%	81%	77%	74%	71%	68%	65%	63%	61%
9	95%	90%	86%	82%	78%	75%	72%	69%	67%	64%	62%
9.5	95%	90%	86%	83%	79%	76%	73%	70%	68%	66%	63%
10	95%	91%	87%	83%	80%	77%	74%	71%	69%	67%	65%

*Greater than 70% N$_2$O administered exceeds the amount able to be delivered by sedation machine.

Liters per minute O$_2$

6	6.5	7	7.5	8	8.5	9	9.5	10
8%	7%	7%	6%	6%	6%	5%	5%	5%
14%	13%	13%	12%	11%	11%	10%	10%	9%
20%	19%	18%	17%	16%	15%	14%	14%	13%
25%	24%	22%	21%	20%	19%	18%	17%	17%
29%	28%	26%	25%	24%	23%	22%	21%	20%
33%	32%	30%	29%	27%	26%	25%	24%	23%
37%	35%	33%	32%	30%	29%	28%	27%	26%
40%	38%	36%	35%	33%	32%	31%	30%	29%
43%	41%	39%	38%	36%	35%	33%	32%	31%
45%	43%	42%	40%	38%	37%	36%	34%	33%
48%	46%	44%	42%	41%	39%	38%	37%	35%
50%	48%	46%	44%	43%	41%	40%	39%	38%
52%	50%	48%	46%	45%	43%	42%	41%	39%
54%	52%	50%	48%	47%	45%	44%	42%	41%
56%	54%	52%	50%	48%	47%	45%	44%	43%
57%	55%	53%	52%	50%	48%	47%	46%	44%
59%	57%	55%	53%	52%	50%	49%	47%	46%
60%	58%	56%	55%	53%	51%	50%	49%	47%
61%	59%	58%	56%	54%	53%	51%	50%	49%
63%	61%	59%	57%	56%	54%	53%	51%	50%

N₂O/O₂ Sedation Record

Date: _____ Patient Name: _____ Age: _____

ASA Classification: I   II   III   IV

Indications for N_2O/O_2: _____

Procedural Date:

	PREOPERATIVE	INTRAOPERATIVE (Moderate Sedation)	POSTOPERATIVE
Blood pressure:	_____	_____	_____
Pulse:	_____	_____	_____
Respiration:	_____	_____	_____
Sp_{O_2} (moderate sedation):	_____	_____	_____

Tidal volume(L/min): _____   Peak % N_2O adm: _____

Postop 100% O_2: _____   minutes

Recovery (pt comments): _____

Adverse Reactions/Comments:

Clinician's signature: _____

Informed Consent for N_2O/O_2 Sedation

I understand that my treatment today will include the procedure of N_2O/O_2 administration. I, _____, have been informed of the purpose of the procedure and how it will benefit my treatment. The procedure has been described to me and I understand how it will be accomplished. I should feel more relaxed and less anxious.

I understand that certain risk(s) may be associated with this procedure, such as headache, dizziness, nausea, and vomiting. Some patients at high levels of N_2O can experience dreaming and hallucinations. I understand the risk(s) associated with this procedure and I further understand the risk(s) that may occur if the procedure is not completed.

I also realize that my doctor must know if I have taken any type of medication or drugs within the past seventy-two (72) hours because these may cause an adverse reaction when N_2O/O_2 is administered. I verify that I have told my doctor about any such medications and drugs.

I have been informed of the alternatives to N_2O/O_2 sedation and their associated risks.

All of my questions and concerns have been satisfactorily answered and addressed.

Therefore, I give my informed consent to the administration of N_2O/O_2 sedation and agree to hold harmless, release, and indemnify agents, servants, students, and employees of the office/clinic of _____ from any and all causes of action, claims, demands, or liability that may arise out of such treatment on behalf of myself, my heirs, my executors, administrators or assigns; or on behalf of my minor child or children or his/her (their) heirs, executors, administrators or assigns.

Signed: _____   Date: _____

Witness: _____   Date: _____

Overview of Administration of N$_2$O/O$_2$ Sedation

1. Inspect all N$_2$O/O$_2$ equipment for proper setup. Periodically check pressure connections with a soap and water solution per manufacturer's recommendations. Inspect the tubing and reservoir bag for cracks or tears.
2. Confirm the adequacy of all scavenging methods to include the vacuum exhaust and ventilation for the area.
3. Review the patient's health history and record vital signs. Obtain informed consent.
4. Activate O$_2$ flow, fit nasal hood or face mask, and establish appropriate tidal volume. Observe reservoir bag.
5. Initiate N$_2$O flow and titrate appropriately while constantly assessing the patient.
6. Upon termination of the N$_2$O, begin a minimum postoperative oxygenation period of 5 minutes.
7. Assess the patient for appropriate recovery. Administer additional O$_2$ if necessary.
8. Document the procedure appropriately in the patient's file (i.e., sedation record).
9. Properly disassemble and disinfect equipment.

Index

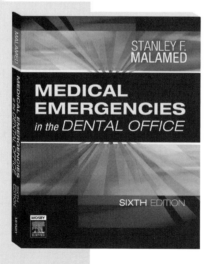